The **Dysphagia** Cookbook

Delicious and Easy Swallowing Recipes for Health, Happiness, and Confidence

Martha McGrew

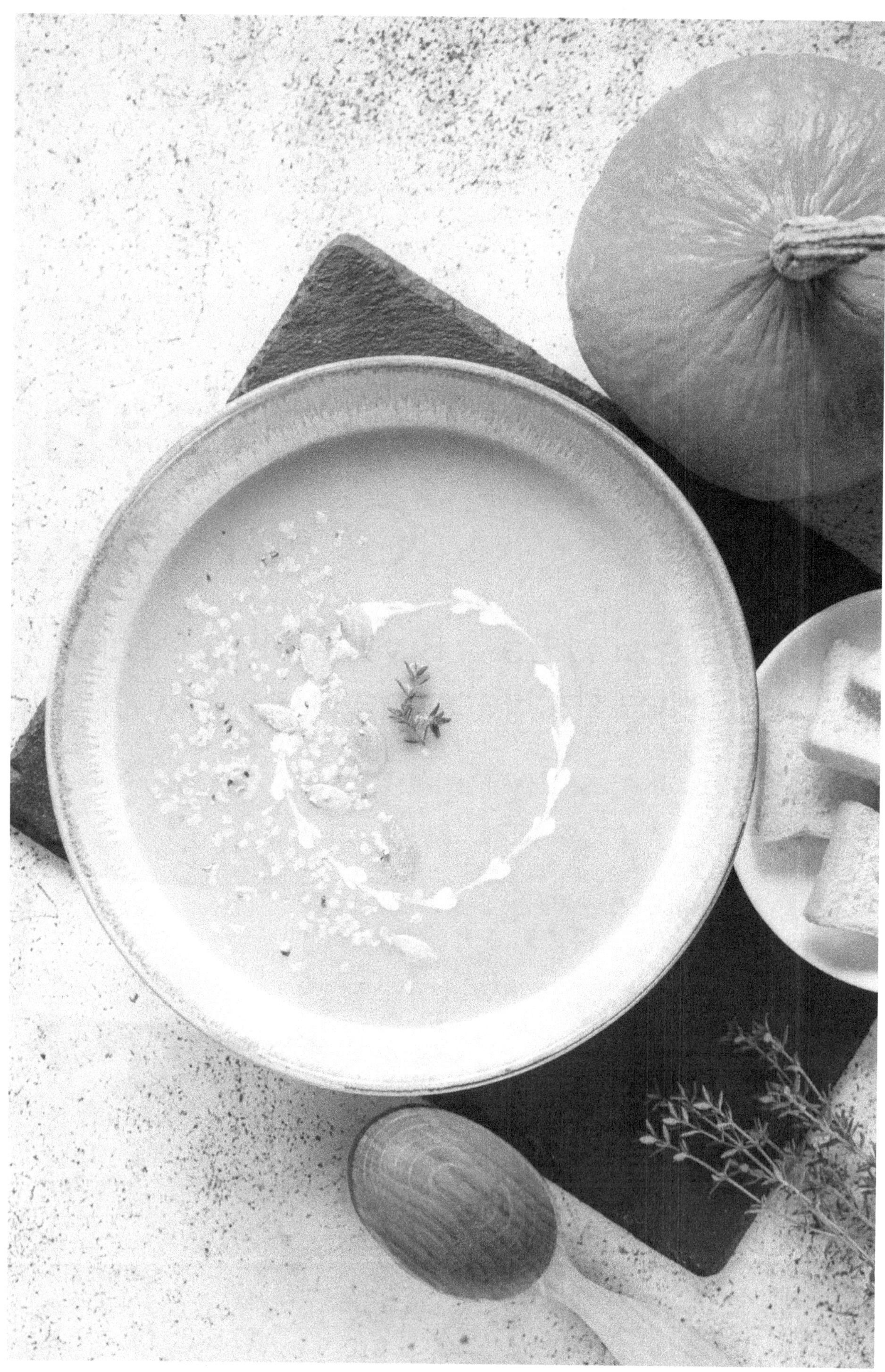

Thank You!

I hope you will enjoy reading it as much as I enjoyed writing it. <u>Your support means the world to me!</u>

If you will find value in these pages, I kindly ask you to consider **leaving an honest review on Amazon.** Your feedback not only helps me improve but also helps other readers discover this book.

BONUS

UNLOCK CULINARY FREEDOM WITH:

"CAREGIVER'S TOOLKIT"

YOUR KEYS TO EASE & NOURISHMENT
AWAIT AT THE END OF THE BOOK!

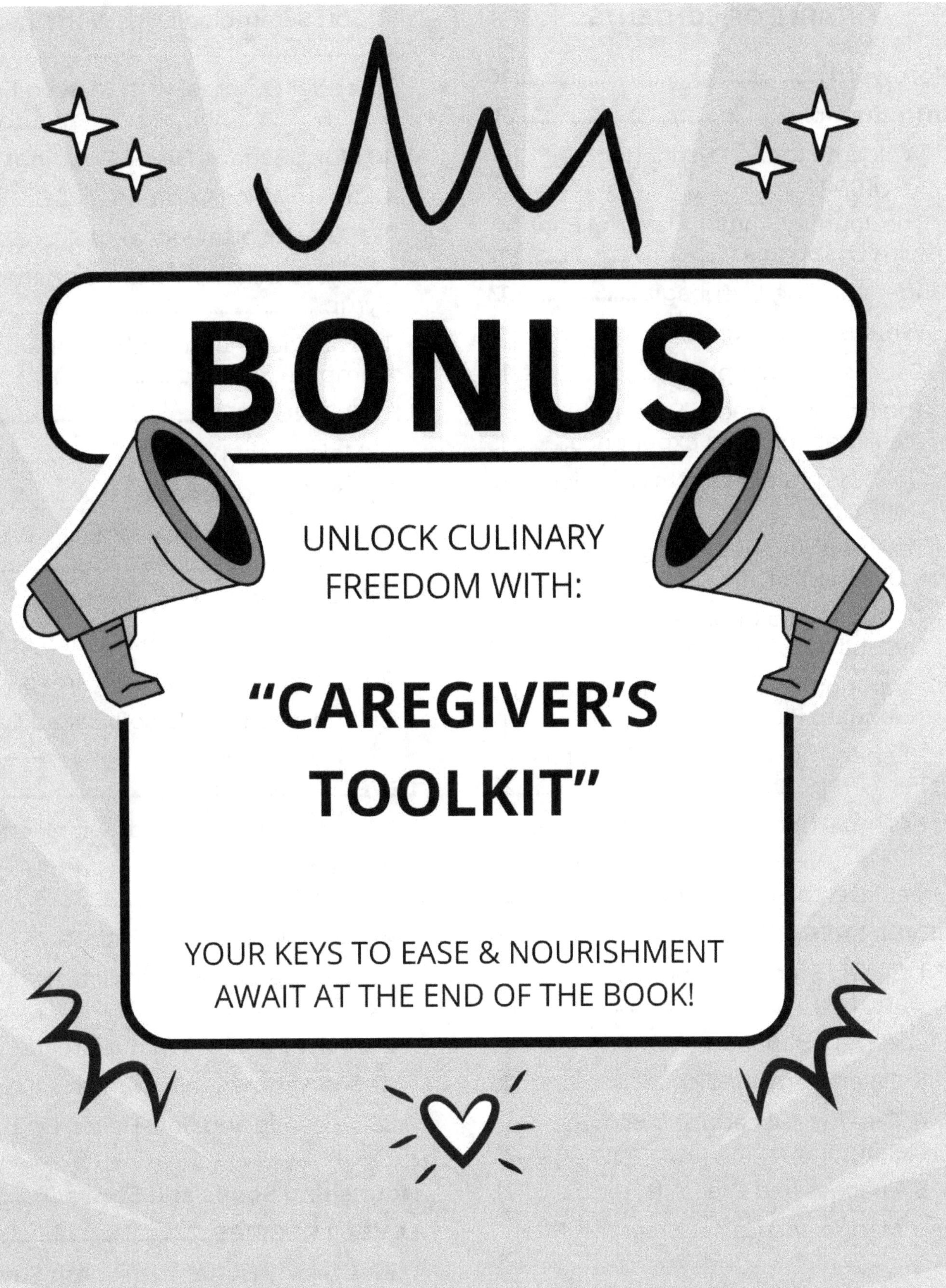

TABLE OF CONTENTS:

Foreword **10**

Introduction **11**

Welcome to the Dysphagia Cookbook...11

The Journey Ahead: Flavorful Eating with Dysphagia 12

Understanding Dysphagia **13**

What is Dysphagia?.................................13

Causes and Symptoms........................14

The Importance of a Safe and Pleasurable Eating Experience............15

How Dysphagia Affects Nutrition and Daily Life 16

Textures: Understanding the Levels in a Dysphagia Diet................................17

Tailored Food Choices for Each Dysphagia Diet Level 18

Hydration and Dysphagia: Ensuring Adequate Fluid Intake 19

Kitchen Tools and Equipment for Easy Prep...20

Essential Cooking Techniques and Tips 21

Breakfasts to Start Your Day **23**

LEVEL 1 RECIPES **24**

1. Classic Smooth Apple-Cinnamon Oatmeal 24

2..Velvety Banana Yogurt Smoothie24

3. Silken Berry Medley 25

4. Creamy Avocado and Spinach Delight 25

5. Peaches and Cream Puree 25

6. Mango and Carrot Breakfast Bliss 26

7. Soothing Pumpkin Pie Porridge ..26

LEVEL 2 RECIPES **27**

8. Soft Scrambled Eggs with Cheddar 27

9.Tender Oatmeal with Stewed Fruit 27

10.Moist Banana Bread Pudding.......28

11.Creamy Rice Pudding 28

12.Fluffy Ricotta Pancakes....................29

13.Soft Poached Pears in Cinnamon Syrup...29

14.Cottage Cheese with Soft Peach Compote 29

LEVEL 3 RECIPES **30**

15.Moist French Toast 30

16.Soft Baked Omelet...........................31

17. Creamy Banana Oatmeal with Pureed Berries 31

18.Creamy Polenta with Cheese 32

19.Soft Pancakes with Maple Syrup..32

20.Avocado Toast on Soft Bread.........33

21.Cinnamon-Apple Soft Baked Bars 33

LEVEL 4 RECIPES..................................**34**

22.Soft Scrambled Eggs with Herbs34

23.Creamy Greek Yogurt with Honey and Soft Fruits...34

24.Tender Vegetable Frittata.............34

25.Cottage Cheese and Soft Peach Bowl 35

26.Moist Banana-Walnut Bread 35

27.Soft Whole Grain Waffles.................36

28. Avocado and Soft-Boiled Egg Toast 36

Nourishing Soups and Stews **37**

LEVEL 1 RECIPES **38**

29. Creamy Butternut Squash Soup38

30. Silky Carrot and Ginger Soup 38

31. Velvety Potato and Leek Soup......39

32. Smooth Tomato Basil Soup 39

33. Pureed Pea and Mint Soup 39

34. Creamy Broccoli Soup......................40

35. Pumpkin and Apple Soup...............41

LEVEL2 RECIPES..**41**

36. Soft Lentil and Vegetable Soup ..41

37. Tender Chicken and Rice Soup ...41

38. Creamy Cauliflower and Cheese Soup...42

39. Soft Split Pea Soup with Ham 43

40. Gentle Beef and Potato Stew 43

41. Soft Barley and Mushroom Soup 44

42. Smooth Pumpkin Bisque 44

LEVEL3 RECIPES **45**

43. Chunky Potato and Leek Soup ..45

44. Tender Chicken Noodle Soup.....45

45. Hearty Minestrone with Soft Vegetables...46

46. Creamy Fish Chowder......................46

47. Soft Beef and Barley Stew 47

48. Butternut Squash and Carrot Soup..47

49. Mildly Spiced Lentil Stew 48

LEVEL4 RECIPES **49**

50. Hearty Vegetable Beef Stew........49

51. Creamy Chicken and Wild Rice Soup..49

52. Tuscan White Bean and Kale Soup 50

53. Tomato Basil Bisque with Soft Mozzarella...50

54. Mushroom and Barley Soup 51

55. Sweet Potato and Corn Chowder 51

56. Savory Pumpkin and Ginger Soup 52

Main Courses......................................**53**

LEVEL 1 RECIPES **54**

57.Smooth Chicken and Vegetable Puree 54

58. Creamy Pureed Fish with Dill......54

59. Velvety Beef and Potato Puree ..55

60. Silken Tofu and Spinach Blend ..55

61. Pureed Turkey with Gravy..............55

62. Savory Lentil and Carrot Puree...56

63. Butternut Squash and Apple Puree 56

LEVEL2 RECIPES..**57**

64. Soft Chicken and Rice Casserole 57

65. Tender Meatloaf with Gravy..........57

66. Moist Salmon Patties......................58

67. Creamy Mashed Potato and Cheese Bake...58

68. Soft Vegetable Risotto....................59

69. Tender Beef Stroganoff...................59

70. Soft-Cooked Chicken and Vegetable Pie..60

LEVEL3 RECIPES..**60**

71. Moist Chicken Parmesan................60

72. Soft Shepherd's Pie 61

73. Tender Baked Fish Fillet...................61

74. Soft-Cooked Pork Chops with Applesauce...62

75. Creamy Tuna and Noodle Casserole...62

76. Soft Roasted Turkey with Gravy.63

77. Slow-Cooked Beef Goulash...........63

LEVEL4 RECIPES **64**

78. Tender Grilled Chicken with Soft Herb Polenta..64

79. Moist Meatballs in Marinara Sauce 64

80. Flaky Baked Salmon with Dill Sauce 65

81. Slow-Cooked Pulled Pork with Soft Rolls 65

82. Soft-Cooked Beef Stroganoff over Egg Noodles 66

83. Baked Lasagna with Soft Cheese Filling 66

84. Creamy Vegetable Curry with Soft Rice 67

Sides and Snacks 68

LEVEL 1 RECIPES 69

85. Smooth Mashed Butternut Squash 69

86. Creamy Pureed Peas 69

87. Velvety Carrot and Ginger Puree 70

88. Silken Pear and Apple Compote 70

89. Smooth Avocado Puree 70

90. Silken Tofu and Berry Compote ..71

91. Creamy Mashed Cauliflower 71

LEVEL2 RECIPES 72

92. Soft-Cooked Mashed Potatoes ...72

93. Tender Steamed Broccoli Puree 72

94. Honeyed Pear Puree 73

95. Soft Baked Apple Slices 73

96. Moist Pumpkin Custard 74

97. Soft Pear and Cottage Cheese ...74

98. Soft Rice Pudding 74

LEVEL3 RECIPES 75

99. Soft-Cooked Carrot and Swede Mash 75

100. Tender Peas and Carrots in Butter 75

101. Moist Zucchini Bread 76

102. Creamy Baked Custard 76

103. Soft Banana Pudding 77

104. Tender Baked Pear Halves 77

105. Fluffy Scrambled Eggs with Cheese 78

LEVEL4 RECIPES 78

106. Soft Baked Apple and Cinnamon Wedges 78

107. Creamy Mashed Sweet Potatoes 79

108. Tender Steamed Green Beans with Almonds 79

109. Moist Banana Mini-Muffins 79

110. Soft-Cooked Pear Compote 80

111. Creamy Rice and Cheese Bake ...80

112. Velvet Zucchini Blend 81

Desserts and Sweet Treats 82

LEVEL 1 RECIPES 83

113. Silky Mango Mousse 83

114. Creamy Vanilla Pudding 83

115. Velvety Chocolate Avocado Pudding 83

116. Smooth Berry Gelatin 84

117. Pumpkin Spice Puree 84

118. Silken Rice Pudding 85

119. Pureed Baked Apple with Cinnamon 85

LEVEL2 RECIPES 86

120. Soft Baked Custard 86

121. Creamy Banana Yogurt Parfait ..86

122. Tender Stewed Fruit Compote .87

123. Moist Carrot Cake Pudding 87

124. Soft Poached Pears in Vanilla Syrup 88

125. Mango and Coconut Rice Pudding 88

126. Rice Pudding with Soft Raisins ..89

LEVEL3 RECIPES 89

127. Soft-Baked Apple Crisp 89

128. Moist Lemon Sponge Cake 90

129. Tender Blueberry Muffins............90

130. Creamy Cheesecake with Soft Fruit Topping 91

131. Fluffy Chocolate Mousse 91

132. Soft Poached Fruit Medley 92

133. Baked Rice Pudding with Soft Raisins...92

LEVEL4 RECIPES 93

134. Soft-Baked Peach Cobbler 93

135. Creamy Banana Bread...................93

136. Tender Fruit Trifle.............................94

137. Fluffy Angel Food Cake with Soft Berry Compote 95

138. Moist Carrot Cake with Cream Cheese Frosting 95

139. Soft Pumpkin Pie 96

140. Creamy Chocolate Pudding.......96

Beverages and Smoothies..................97

LEVEL 1 RECIPES 98

141. Thickened Apple Juice 98

142. Creamy Vanilla Thickened Milkshake 98

143. Smooth Berry Puree Smoothie 98

144. Velvety Chocolate Thickened Beverage..98

145. Thickened Mango Nectar............99

LEVEL2 RECIPES.................................... 99

146. Creamy Banana Smoothie 99

147. Soft Berry Yogurt Drink................100

148. Gentle Peach and Pear Nectar 100

149. Smooth Avocado and Honey Shake...100

LEVEL3 RECIPES...................................101

150. Tender Peach Smoothie..............101

151. Soft Mixed Berry Compote Drink 101

152. Creamy Oatmeal and Banana Shake...102

153. Soft Apple and Cinnamon Swirl 102

154. Mildly Chunky Mango Lassi.......102

LEVEL4 RECIPES 103

155. Gentle Pear and Ginger Smoothie..103

156. Soft Blueberry and Yogurt Drink 103

157. Creamy Avocado-Cocoa Smoothie..103

158. Strawberry-Banana Swirl 104

159. Melon and Mint Refresher..........104

Foreword

As a healthcare professional who has spent years navigating the challenging waters of dysphagia management, I am profoundly aware of the obstacles faced by individuals who struggle with swallowing disorders. The quest for nourishment, once a source of pleasure, can become a source of anxiety and frustration for patients and caregivers alike. It is with this understanding and a heartfelt commitment to improving the lives of those affected that I endorse the content presented in this "Dysphagia Cookbook."

The Unseen Journey of a Meal

The act of swallowing is an intricate ballet of muscles and reflexes that most of us take for granted. However, for someone with dysphagia, each meal is a journey through a path strewn with hurdles. Have you ever pondered the hidden struggle behind each effortless swallow? This cookbook not only ponders it but also presents a roadmap to transform this journey from a path of perils to one of simple pleasures.

Crafted with Care and Expertise

This collection of recipes and guidelines is a testament to the thoughtful and meticulous approach required to cater to the needs of those with swallowing difficulties. Each recipe in this cookbook has been crafted with care, ensuring that:

- **Safety is paramount:** Textures are modified and tested for ease of swallowing.
- **Nutrition is uncompromised:** There is a diligent effort to ensure that the joy of eating does not come at the cost of nutritional adequacy.
- **Flavor takes the forefront:** The misconception that texture-modified foods are unpalatable is dispelled with every savory bite recommended in this book.

A Collaborative Symphony

In creating this cookbook, there has been a symphony of collaboration between dietitians, speech therapists, and culinary experts. This multidisciplinary approach guarantees that the recommendations are not only safe and practical but also delightful to the palate.

Empowerment Through Education

Beyond recipes, this book serves as an educational tool, empowering individuals and their families with the knowledge to understand dysphagia better and tackle it head-on. The strategies and tips provided are invaluable, offering readers a sense of autonomy and control in their dietary choices.

As we turn each page of this Dysphagia Cookbook, we uncover more than just recipes; we unveil a new chapter in the culinary experiences for individuals with dysphagia. The respect and understanding for the condition echoed through these pages affirm my endorsement of this book's content. May it be a source of inspiration, comfort, and enjoyment for those who need it most.

Introduction

Dear Reader,

Welcome to a culinary journey tailored to meet the needs of those navigating the intricate challenges of dysphagia. Whether you are someone who experiences difficulty swallowing, a caregiver seeking to provide nutritious and appetizing meals, or a healthcare professional looking for reliable resources, this cookbook is for you.

Swallowing is a gift most of us never think to unwrap, but for those who face dysphagia, each meal can feel like solving a complex puzzle. This cookbook is crafted to transform that puzzle into a picture of possibility and enjoyment, where every meal becomes an opportunity for nourishment and pleasure.

A Safe Harbor in the Culinary Sea
Navigating the dietary restrictions of dysphagia can often feel like sailing in uncharted waters. The "Dysphagia Cookbook" serves as your compass, guiding you towards safe and delectable harbors. It is your trusty mate in the galley, ensuring that each dish you prepare is not only safe to consume but also a celebration of taste.

Beyond Just Recipes
This book is not just a collection of recipes; it's a beacon of hope and a testament to the creativity that can flourish within the parameters of dietary restrictions. Here, you will find:

- A diverse palette of flavors that honor both classic and innovative cuisine.
- Guidance on how to modify textures without compromising on the joy of eating.
- Nutritional advice to support the overall well-being of those with dysphagia.
- We invite you to flip through these pages with an open mind and a willing palate. Within this cookbook, you will discover that the challenges of dysphagia do not mark the end of delightful eating, but rather the beginning of a new culinary adventure.

You Are Not Alone
Remember, you are part of a community that understands your journey. This cookbook is a bridge connecting you to countless others who share your experiences. Together, we can turn each meal into a cherished moment, full of flavor and joy.

So, let's roll up our sleeves, gather our ingredients, and embark on this flavorful quest. Here's to the satisfaction of a well-prepared meal that is both safe and scrumptious!

Embarking on the journey of eating with dysphagia can feel like navigating a new world—a world where the rules of eating are rewritten. But within these pages lies a map to a destination teeming with rich flavors, safe textures, and the joy of mealtime once again. This is not merely about eating; it's about relishing life one spoonful at a time.

Discover a Spectrum of Flavors

The "Dysphagia Cookbook" is your culinary companion, promising that a diagnosis does not define your diet. We'll explore together how:

- **Spices and herbs** can paint bold strokes of flavor across the canvas of soft textures.
- **Techniques like roasting or caramelizing** can unlock a treasure trove of taste, turning the simple into the sublime.
- **Variety remains the spice of life**, with recipes ranging from hearty soups to delectable desserts, ensuring that your palate never wearers.

Texture Meets Technique

A mastery of texture is critical in the art of dysphagia cuisine. You will learn to craft dishes that are not only safe but also inviting, using:

- **Thickening** agents that bring consistency without muting flavor.
- **Blending** methods that preserve the essence of the ingredient's natural taste.
- **Layering flavors** to create dishes that are as appealing to the eye as they are to the tongue.

Empowerment Through Education

The knowledge you'll gain here goes beyond recipes. It's about empowering you with the skills to adapt your favorite meals to meet your needs or the needs of those you care for. The "Dysphagia Cookbook" equips you with:

- **Tips and tricks** for meal planning and preparation.
- **Advice on kitchen tools** that can make cooking for dysphagia simpler and more efficient.
- **Nutritional guidance** to ensure that every meal contributes to overall health and well-being.

As you turn each page, you are taking a step towards reclaiming the pleasure of eating. The "Dysphagia Cookbook" is your guide, your friend, and your inspiration. Together, let's savor the journey ahead, where every meal is an adventure waiting to be cherished.

Welcome to flavorful eating with dysphagia. Welcome to a world of possibility.

Understanding Dysphagia

Dysphagia is a medical term that describes a condition where individuals experience difficulty in swallowing. It may be due to a range of underlying health issues, affecting any part of the swallowing process—from the initial action of chewing food to the movement of that food down the esophagus and into the stomach.

The Swallowing Process
To appreciate the complexity of dysphagia, it's important to understand what a normal swallowing process entails. Swallowing is a dynamic action that involves around 50 pairs of muscles and many nerves, working in concert to move food from the mouth to the stomach safely. This process is divided into three stages:

1. **Oral Phase:** The preparation of food in the mouth, chewing it to the right texture, and forming it into a ball (bolus) ready for swallowing.
2. **Pharyngeal Phase:** The beginning of the swallow and the movement of the bolus into the throat.
3. **Esophageal Phase:** The bolus transits down the esophagus and into the stomach.

Types of Dysphagia
Dysphagia can be classified based on where the swallowing problem occurs:

- **Oropharyngeal Dysphagia:** Issues in the mouth and throat, often related to neurological problems, muscular disorders, or structural abnormalities.
- **Esophageal Dysphagia:** Issues in the esophagus, which may be caused by esophageal muscle problems, blockages, or irritation.

Symptoms and Complications
The experience of dysphagia can range from mild difficulty to a complete inability to swallow. Symptoms may include coughing or choking when eating or drinking, sensation of food stuck in the throat, recurrent pneumonia, weight loss, and dehydration. If left unmanaged, dysphagia can lead to serious complications, including malnutrition and respiratory problems.

Managing Dysphagia
Managing dysphagia often involves a team approach, including medical doctors, speech-language pathologists, dietitians, and occupational therapists. Treatment and management strategies can include swallowing therapy, dietary modifications, and, in some cases, medical or surgical intervention.

In the context of dietary modifications, texture-modified foods, and thickened liquids play a significant role. They are easier to swallow and reduce the risk of choking and aspiration (food or liquid entering the airway), which is where the "Dysphagia Cookbook" can be an invaluable resource.

As we delve deeper into the world of dysphagia, understanding its potential causes and recognizing its symptoms becomes crucial. This knowledge not only aids in managing the condition but also empowers those affected to seek appropriate care and make informed decisions about their health and diet.

Causes of Dysphagia
Dysphagia can be caused by a wide array of health conditions, each affecting the swallowing process in different ways. Some common causes include:

- **Neurological Disorders:** Conditions like stroke, Parkinson's disease, multiple sclerosis, and cerebral palsy can affect the nerves that control swallowing muscles.
- **Head and Neck Cancers:** Tumors in the mouth, throat, or esophagus can physically obstruct the passage of food or weaken the muscles involved in swallowing.
- **Muscular Disorders:** Issues such as muscular dystrophy can weaken the muscles needed for effective swallowing.
- **Gastroesophageal Reflux Disease (GERD):** Chronic acid reflux can irritate and damage the lining of the esophagus, leading to swallowing difficulties.
- **Aging:** Natural aging can result in a gradual decline in the strength and coordination of swallowing muscles.

Symptoms of Dysphagia
The symptoms associated with dysphagia may vary depending on the underlying cause and the severity of the condition. Some common symptoms include:

- **Difficulty Initiating Swallow:** A feeling that it takes more effort to start swallowing.
- **Coughing or Choking:** This can happen during or after eating, indicating that food is going down the wrong way.
- **Sensation of Food Being Stuck:** A persistent feeling that food is lodged in the throat or chest after swallowing.
- **Unexplained Weight Loss:** Due to the difficulty of consuming enough calories.
- **Avoidance of Certain Foods or Liquids:** Preferring certain textures or temperatures that are easier to swallow.
- **Recurrent Pneumonia:** Caused by food particles entering the lungs, known as aspiration pneumonia.
- **Regurgitation:** Food coming back up after swallowing.

Recognizing these symptoms early and consulting with healthcare professionals can lead to better management strategies and reduce the risk of complications. Adjusting the texture and consistency of food, as well as incorporating therapeutic techniques can significantly improve the safety and enjoyment of eating for individuals with dysphagia.

For those with dysphagia, the significance of a safe and pleasurable eating experience cannot be overstated. It is a balancing act that marries the joy of taste with the necessity of nutrition, ensuring that the act of eating supports both the body and the spirit.

Safety: The First Priority
Before the pleasures of flavor come into play, safety takes precedence. Here's why:

- **Preventing Aspiration:** Safe swallowing practices reduce the risk of food or liquid entering the lungs, which can lead to aspiration pneumonia.
- **Avoiding Malnutrition:** Ensuring that the food consumed is easy to swallow encourages regular eating and helps prevent malnutrition and dehydration.

The Role of Pleasure in Eating
Once safety is assured, the focus turns to the experience of eating, which is vital for several reasons:

- **Psychological Well-being:** Enjoying food can significantly enhance the quality of life, providing comfort and pleasure in daily routines.
- **Social Inclusion:** Meals are often social events. Being able to participate can reduce feelings of isolation and improve overall happiness.
- **Motivation to Eat:** Tasty food encourages regular eating, which is essential for maintaining strength and health.

Crafting a Safe and Enjoyable Meal
So how do we craft meals that are both safe and enjoyable? It requires a thoughtful approach:

- **Texture Modification:** Adjusting the texture of food to meet the individual's needs without compromising on taste.
- **Flavor Enhancement:** Employing a variety of herbs, spices, and cooking techniques to enrich the flavor profile of soft or pureed foods.
- **Visual Appeal:** Presenting food in an appealing way to stimulate appetite and make meals more inviting.
- **Experimentation and Variety:** Offering a diverse range of dishes to provide a balanced diet and prevent menu fatigue.

The "Dysphagia Cookbook" and Beyond
This book serves as a foundational tool for those seeking to navigate the complexities of cooking for dysphagia. It's a starting point for:

- **Exploring New Recipes:** Trying out tailored recipes that are specifically designed to be both safe and flavorful.
- **Learning Techniques:** Gaining skills in preparing meals that align with the necessary precautions for dysphagia.

- **Sharing with Others:** Using the recipes and tips within to share the joy of eating with friends and family, regardless of their swallowing abilities.

Eating is one of life's great joys and a fundamental human experience. For individuals with dysphagia, achieving a safe and pleasurable eating experience is essential for physical health and emotional satisfaction. Through the guidance offered in the "Dysphagia Cookbook," readers will learn that a diagnosis of dysphagia is not an end to enjoyable eating, but rather the start of a new culinary journey that can be as rich and flavorful as ever before.

How Dysphagia Affects Nutrition and Daily Life

Dysphagia can have far-reaching effects on an individual's health and day-to-day living. It is not just a challenge during mealtimes; its impact spills over into overall nutrition, hydration, and quality of life.

Nutritional Challenges

When it becomes difficult to swallow, the intake of adequate nutrients and fluids can become a serious concern:

- **Limited Food Choices:** Those with dysphagia may avoid a variety of foods, leading to a restricted diet that lacks essential nutrients.
- **Risk of Malnutrition:** Difficulty with eating can result in consuming fewer calories, proteins, and other nutrients needed for energy and repair of body tissues.
- **Dehydration Risk:** Similarly, if drinking is a challenge, the risk of dehydration increases, which can lead to numerous health issues.

Impact on Daily Life

Dysphagia can transform routine activities into challenging tasks, influencing several aspects of daily living:

- **Extended Meal Times:** Eating with dysphagia often requires more time, affecting schedules and daily routines.
- **Social Implications:** Dining is a social event, and dysphagia can lead to embarrassment or anxiety around eating with others.
- **Emotional Effects:** The stress of dealing with dysphagia can lead to feelings of isolation, frustration, and depression.

Ensuring Adequate Nutrition

Addressing the nutritional needs of someone with dysphagia involves careful planning:

- **Balanced Meals:** Ensuring that each meal contains the right balance of carbohydrates, proteins, fats, vitamins, and minerals.
- **Supplemental Nutrition:** Sometimes, supplements are necessary to provide nutrients that cannot be consumed in sufficient quantities through regular meals.

- **Hydration Strategies:** Implementing creative ways to maintain hydration, such as offering flavored waters, gels, or foods with high water content.

Improving Quality of Life

With thoughtful strategies, the quality of life for those with dysphagia can be greatly enhanced:

- **Tailored Eating Aids:** Utilizing specially designed utensils, cups, and plates to make eating easier and more efficient.
- **Adaptive Cooking:** The "Dysphagia Cookbook" offers recipes and techniques to prepare enjoyable and nutritious meals that meet the unique needs of those with dysphagia.
- **Professional Support:** Speech and language therapists can provide exercises and strategies to improve swallowing ability, while dietitians can assist in creating an appropriate meal plan.

Dysphagia is more than just a physical ailment—it is a condition that touches every part of life. It requires a comprehensive approach to maintain not just nutritional health, but also the joy and community that come with eating. Through resources like the "Dysphagia Cookbook," individuals with dysphagia and their caregivers are empowered with the knowledge and tools to mitigate the condition's impact, ensuring that each meal is a step towards nourishment and normalcy.

Textures: Understanding the Levels in a Dysphagia Diet

Texture plays a pivotal role in the dysphagia diet, providing structure and safety for those with swallowing difficulties. The diet is categorized into different texture levels, each designed to match the swallowing capabilities of the individual. Let's break down what each texture level means in the dysphagia diet.

Level 1: Pureed (Homogenous)

- **Characteristics:** Smooth, pudding-like, no lumps.
- **Preparation Tips:** Foods should be blended to a consistent texture and may require a thickening agent to achieve the right consistency.
- **Examples:** Pureed fruits, vegetables, meats, and cooked cereals.

Level 2: Mechanically Altered (Soft)

- **Characteristics:** Moist, cohesive, and slightly thicker than pureed, easily formed into a bolus.
- **Preparation Tips:** Foods need to be well-cooked and can be chopped, ground, or mashed.
- **Examples:** Soft flaked fish, ripe banana, or mashed potatoes.

Level 3: Advanced

- **Characteristics:** Near-normal texture but not hard, sticky, or crunchy.
- **Preparation Tips:** Avoid skins, seeds, and anything that requires bolting or hard chewing.

- **Examples:** Moist tender meats, soft-cooked vegetables, and soft ripe fruit.

Level 4: Regular

- **Characteristics:** All textures are allowed except for the most challenging ones like tough meats, hard fruits and vegetables, and very dry or crumbly textures.
- **Preparation Tips:** Ensure foods are cooked to be tender and are cut into bite-sized pieces.
- **Examples:** A full variety of foods, barring exclusions like nuts, seeds, and dry crackers.

A Note to the Reader:
Remember, transitioning between texture levels should always be done under the guidance of a healthcare professional. Only they can adequately assess the progression and ensure the dysphagia diet's safety and nutritional adequacy for the individual.

Key Takeaway:
The varying texture levels in a dysphagia diet serve to protect against choking and aspiration while ensuring nutritional needs are met. Each level is designed to provide a satisfying meal experience while catering to the specific requirements of the individual's swallowing ability. Whether one is starting with pureed foods or advancing to more regular textures, the "Dysphagia Cookbook" is a resourceful guide for navigating these waters with confidence and care.

Tailored Food Choices for Each Dysphagia Diet Level

Crafting a menu for someone with dysphagia involves a delicate balance of texture and nutrition. Here's a guide to appropriate food choices for each level of the dysphagia diet.

Level 1: Pureed Consistency
At this initial stage, food must be smooth and free from lumps:

- **Fruits and Vegetables:** Pureed applesauce, smooth carrot puree, or ripe banana mashed to a fine consistency.
- **Proteins:** Blended lean meats, pureed beans, or smooth cottage cheese.
- **Grains:** Pureed oatmeal, cream of wheat, or finely ground and moistened rice.
- **Dairy:** Smooth yogurts and pureed soft cheeses.

Level 2: Soft and Well-Cooked
Soft and well-cooked options that require minimal chewing include:

- **Fruits and Vegetables:** Soft steamed vegetables like broccoli or squash, and soft fruits like canned peaches or ripe avocado.
- **Proteins:** Soft fish, finely minced chicken, or scrambled eggs.
- **Grains:** Soft pasta, moistened bread, or soft pancakes.
- **Dairy:** Creamy ricotta cheese or a smooth milkshake.

Level 3: Advanced Textures
Foods at this stage are nearly normal but still easy to chew and swallow:

- **Fruits and Vegetables:** Ripe bananas, cooked fruit compotes, and steamed vegetables cut into small, manageable pieces.
- **Proteins:** Tender meatballs, flaked fish, or moistened baked chicken.
- **Grains:** Moist cake, soft bread without crusts, or tender rice.
- **Dairy:** Custards or soft, non-crusty cheese like Brie.

Level 4: Regular Diet with Modifications
A broader range of foods is allowed, avoiding only the most challenging textures:

- **Fruits and Vegetables: Most** cooked vegetables and ripe fruits, except for those with skins and seeds.
- **Proteins:** All tender-cooked meats and fish, avoiding dry, tough cuts.
- **Grains:** Most cooked grains, soft tortillas, and muffins without nuts or seeds.
- **Dairy:** All dairy products are generally safe, barring any mix-ins like nuts.

Each dysphagia diet level has a spectrum of suitable foods designed to ensure safety and enjoyment. The "Dysphagia Cookbook" provides a wide variety of recipes tailored to these levels, making it possible to enjoy a range of flavors and dishes while adhering to the necessary dietary restrictions. It's about turning necessity into an opportunity for culinary creativity, ensuring those with dysphagia have a delightful and nutritious eating experience.

Note to the Reader:
While the "Dysphagia Cookbook" offers a rich palette of food choices tailored to different levels of swallowing difficulties, it is crucial to remember that each individual's needs are unique. **Before embarking on any of the diet levels outlined above, please consult with a healthcare professional or a registered dietitian.** They can provide a thorough assessment and determine which level of the dysphagia diet is appropriate for you or your loved one. Moreover, they may offer additional personalized recommendations to address specific nutritional needs and ensure that the diet is safe, effective, and enjoyable. Always let the guidance of a medical professional illuminate your path to the right diet choice.

Hydration and Dysphagia: Ensuring Adequate Fluid Intake

Maintaining proper hydration is a critical aspect of health, especially for individuals with dysphagia. The challenge of swallowing liquids safely can increase the risk of dehydration, making it essential to understand and apply strategies for adequate fluid intake.

Proper hydration is not just a matter of quenching thirst—it's vital for bodily functions, including digestion, nutrient transportation, and temperature regulation. It also helps prevent complications like urinary tract infections and constipation, contributing to overall well-being.

For those with dysphagia, beverages often need to be thickened to the appropriate consistency to prevent aspiration. This modification ensures that liquids move through the throat safely, and the consistency of these thickened liquids varies from nectar-like to honey-like, or even pudding-like, depending on the severity of dysphagia. It's important to provide fluids throughout the day, not just at meal times, to ensure a consistent intake.

Getting creative with hydration can also make a significant difference. Flavored gelatins are a fun and appealing way to increase fluids and can be modified to achieve the necessary thickness. Incorporating hydrating foods such as watermelon or pureed soups into the diet is another effective strategy. Monitoring how much liquid is consumed daily can also help reach hydration goals.

It is essential to tailor hydration strategies to the individual's dysphagia level and personal needs, which is best done under the guidance of a healthcare professional. They can offer personalized recommendations and help to incorporate effective hydration methods into daily routines.

In summary, hydration is a key component of managing dysphagia effectively. With the right adjustments and continuous attention to fluid intake, individuals with dysphagia can stay hydrated and healthy. The "Dysphagia Cookbook" not only provides recipes for nutritious and safe-to-swallow meals but also offers inventive ways to ensure that hydration is a delicious and integral part of the daily diet.

Kitchen Tools and Equipment for Easy Prep

When preparing meals for a dysphagia diet, having the right kitchen tools and equipment can transform the experience from a challenging chore to a smooth and efficient process. Not only do these tools make meal prep easier, but they also help ensure that meals meet the necessary texture requirements for safe swallowing.

A food processor is indispensable in the dysphagia kitchen. It can puree fruits, vegetables, and meats to the perfect consistency. Hand blenders are also excellent for pureeing soups and sauces directly in the pot. They're a convenient option for quick tasks without the cleanup required for larger appliances.

Next, a quality blender is essential, especially one that can handle a variety of textures, from grinding dry foods to blending liquids. High-speed blenders are particularly effective for creating smooth, lump-free purees.

A set of mesh strainers of various sizes is beneficial when aiming for the smoothest textures. These can remove any fibrous bits or seeds that might disrupt the uniformity of a puree. For thicker consistencies, a potato ricer can be used to achieve a fine, even mash, ideal for advanced texture levels.

Measuring cups and spoons are necessary to ensure the precise addition of thickeners for liquids, which must be consistent to maintain the prescribed diet level. Digital kitchen scales can help with measuring portions, crucial for those who need to monitor their nutritional intake closely.

Lastly, silicone molds can be a fun addition to the kitchen, allowing you to set purees into shapes, which can be more appealing and add a touch of creativity to meal presentation.

These tools are designed to simplify meal prep, but it's important to prioritize safety and ease of use. Kitchen tools that are easy to handle, clean, and store will be the most beneficial in the long run, making the daily routine of preparing a dysphagia diet as straightforward as possible.

Key Takeaway:
The right kitchen tools can significantly ease the preparation of a dysphagia diet, ensuring meals are safe, nutritious, and appealing. Investing in a few key pieces of equipment can save time, reduce stress, and enhance the overall cooking and eating experience for both the cook and the individual with dysphagia. The "Dysphagia Cookbook" not only guides you through the culinary process with tailored recipes but also through the kitchen setup that makes preparation a breeze.

Essential Cooking Techniques and Tips

Crafting meals for a dysphagia diet calls for specific cooking techniques to ensure dishes are not only safe and easy to swallow but also delicious and nourishing. These methods are designed to maintain nutritional value while achieving the right consistency that's required for different levels of dysphagia.

Steaming is a gentle way to cook foods, preserving their nutrients and natural flavors. It's particularly effective for vegetables and fish, making them soft enough to puree or mash to the needed texture. The added moisture from steaming can also help in achieving a smoother consistency in pureed foods.

Slow cooking is another invaluable technique. By using a slow cooker, meats and vegetables can be cooked at a low temperature over several hours, which can make them tender and perfect for pureeing without a significant loss of flavor.

Poaching is an ideal method for poultry and fish. Cooking at a low temperature in a flavorful liquid not only imparts taste but also ensures the meat remains moist and tender, ideal for those on a dysphagia diet who need soft, easily mashable proteins.

When it comes to **thickening soups or stews**, a roux made from a little butter and flour can be a useful technique, as it allows for a smooth consistency without lumps. For those who need to avoid gluten, cornstarch or a gluten-free flour blend can be effective alternatives.

Pureeing requires attention to detail to achieve the correct consistency. Always start by adding a small amount of liquid to the food processor when pureeing and increase as needed to prevent the mixture from becoming too thin. Also, remember to scrape down the sides of the blender or processor frequently to ensure an even texture without lumps.

In addition to these techniques, here are some general tips that can help in preparing dysphagia-friendly meals:

- **Temperature Matters:** Ensure foods are not too hot or too cold, as extreme temperatures can be uncomfortable or even harmful to a sensitive throat.
- **Flavor is Key:** Just because food is pureed doesn't mean it should be bland. Use herbs, spices, and flavorful broths to enhance taste.
- **Safety First:** Test the consistency of pureed foods before serving to ensure they meet the necessary safety requirements for swallowing.

By incorporating these cooking techniques and tips, meals can be prepared that are safe, nutritious, and enjoyable for those with dysphagia. The "Dysphagia Cookbook" not only includes a range of recipes that utilize these methods but also offers guidance to help caretakers and individuals adapt to this cooking style with confidence and ease.

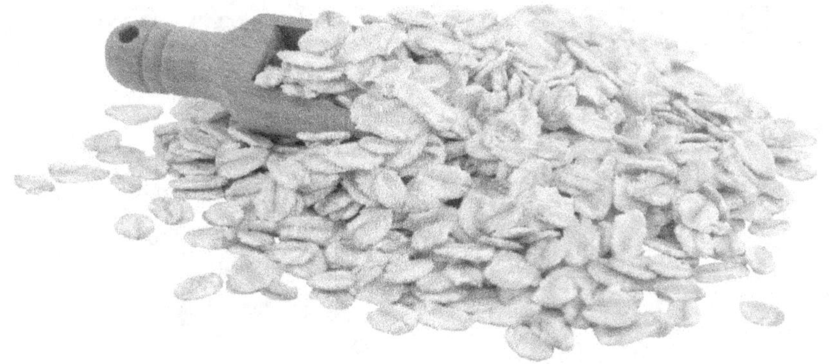

Breakfasts to Start Your Day

They say breakfast is the most important meal of the day, and this holds especially true for those managing swallowing difficulties. This section is dedicated to starting your day on the right note, with meals that are both safe to swallow and a joy to eat.

In these pages, you'll discover a range of breakfast options tailored to various dysphagia diet levels. From smooth, velvety purees to soft, moist meals that are easy to chew and swallow, there's something for everyone. We understand the importance of a good, hearty breakfast in setting the tone for the day, and our recipes are designed to provide the necessary energy and nutrition.

For those on a Pureed Diet (Level 1), we offer smoothie bowls, finely pureed fruits, and creamy oatmeal dishes, ensuring that each spoonful is packed with flavor and nutrients, yet easy and safe to swallow.

For individuals at the Soft and Well-Cooked level (Level 2), the section expands to include gently cooked eggs, soft pancakes, and moist quick bread, providing a bit more texture while still focusing on ease of swallowing.

As we move to Advanced Textures (Level 3), you'll find recipes for soft yet more substantial items like tender French toast and moist scrambled eggs, offering a semblance of normalcy with a mindful approach to texture.

Finally, for those on the **Regular Diet with Modifications (Level 4),** the section includes a broader variety of breakfast foods, such as omelets and soft breakfast sandwiches, ensuring they are prepared in a way that is still mindful of the dysphagia diet requirements.

Every recipe in this section is accompanied by tips on how to modify them for different levels of dysphagia, ensuring that you can adapt them as needed. Whether you're craving something sweet or savory, light or hearty, this section is designed to provide a fulfilling start to your day.

Breakfast is more than just a meal; it's a morning ritual that sets the pace for the hours ahead. With the "Dysphagia Cookbook," you can reclaim the joy of this essential meal, ensuring each morning is greeted with taste, nutrition, and safety in mind.

LEVEL 1 RECIPES

1. Classic Smooth Apple-Cinnamon Oatmeal

Preparation Time: 10 minutes | Cooking Time: 20 minutes

Ingredients:

- 1/2 cup finely ground rolled oats
- 1 cup water or milk (for cooking)
- 1/2 cup apple puree (smooth, no chunks)
- 1/4 teaspoon ground cinnamon
- 1 tablespoon honey or maple syrup (optional)
- Pinch of salt

Instructions:

1. In a saucepan, combine the finely ground oats and water or milk. Stir continuously to prevent lumps.
2. Cook over medium heat until the mixture starts to thicken, about 5-7 minutes.
3. Reduce the heat to low. Add the apple puree, ground cinnamon, honey/maple syrup (if using), and a pinch of salt. Mix well.
4. Continue to cook for another 5-8 minutes, stirring frequently, until the oatmeal reaches a very smooth, almost paste-like consistency.
5. Remove from heat and let it cool slightly. The oatmeal should be smooth and easily swallowable, with no chunks or pieces.

Nutritional Data:

Calories: 290 | Protein: 15g | Carbs: 8g | Fat: 23g | Fiber: 2g | Sugar: 4g

2..Velvety Banana Yogurt Smoothie

Preparation Time: 5 minutes | Cooking Time: 0 minutes

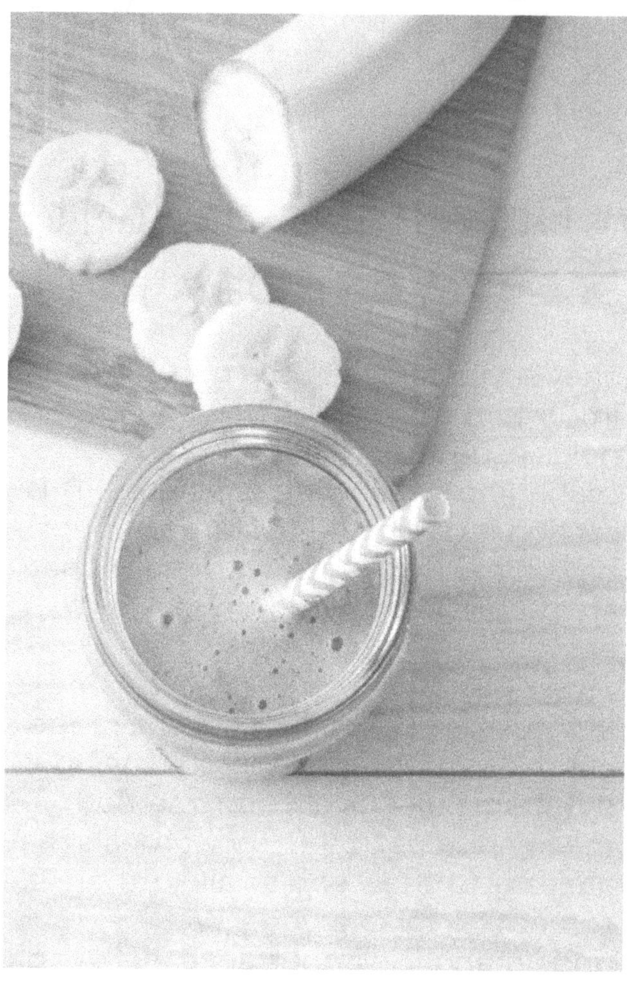

Ingredients:

- 1 ripe banana
- 1/2 cup plain Greek yogurt
- 1/2 cup almond milk or preferred milk
- 1 tablespoon honey or maple syrup (optional)
- A pinch of cinnamon (optional)

Instructions:

1. Peel the banana and cut it into small pieces.
2. Place the banana pieces, Greek yogurt, almond milk,

honey/maple syrup (if using), and cinnamon (if using) in a blender.
3. Blend on high speed until the mixture is completely smooth and has a uniform consistency.
4. Pour the smoothie into a glass. If necessary, you can strain it to ensure it's completely free of lumps.

Nutritional Data:
Calories: 190 | Protein: 8g | Carbs: 34g | Fat: 2g | Fiber: 3g | Sugar: 21g

3. Silken Berry Medley

Preparation Time: 10 minutes | Cooking Time: 0 minutes

Ingredients:

- 1/2 cup mixed berries (like strawberries, raspberries, blueberries) - fresh or frozen
- 1/2 cup Greek yogurt
- 2 tablespoons honey or maple syrup
- 1/4 cup apple juice or water

Instructions:

1. If using frozen berries, thaw them beforehand.
2. Blend the berries, Greek yogurt, honey/maple syrup, and apple juice in a blender until completely smooth.
3. Strain the mixture through a fine mesh to remove any seeds or skin fragments, ensuring a silky texture.

Nutritional Data:
Calories: 200 | Protein: 10g | Carbs: 36g | Fat: 2g | Fiber: 4g | Sugar: 28g

4. Creamy Avocado and Spinach Delight

Preparation Time: 10 minutes | Cooking Time: 0 minutes

Ingredients:

- 1/2 ripe avocado
- 1/2 cup spinach leaves, washed and stems removed
- 1/2 cup Greek yogurt
- 1 tablespoon lemon juice
- Salt and pepper to taste

Instructions:

1. Blend the avocado, spinach, Greek yogurt, and lemon juice in a blender until the mixture is completely smooth.
2. Season with salt and pepper, and blend again to mix well.
3. Strain the mixture if necessary to ensure it is lump-free and smooth.

Nutritional Data:
Calories: 220 | Protein: 9g | Carbs: 12g | Fat: 17g | Fiber: 7g | Sugar: 2g

5. Peaches and Cream Puree

Preparation Time: 5 minutes | Cooking Time: 5 minutes

Ingredients:

- 1 ripe peach, peeled and pitted
- 1/2 cup Greek yogurt
- 1 tablespoon honey or maple syrup
- A pinch of cinnamon (optional)

Instructions:

1. Dice the peach into small pieces.
2. In a small saucepan, cook the peach over medium heat until it becomes soft, about 5 minutes.
3. Allow the peach to cool slightly, then blend it with Greek yogurt and honey/maple syrup until completely smooth.
4. Add a pinch of cinnamon for flavor if desired, and blend again.

Nutritional Data:
Calories: 180 | Protein: 10g | Carbs: 31g | Fat: 2g | Fiber: 2g | Sugar: 28g

6. Mango and Carrot Breakfast Bliss

Preparation Time: 5 minutes | Cooking Time: 10 minutes

Ingredients:

- 1/2 ripe mango, peeled and pitted
- 1/2 cup carrot juice
- 1/2 cup Greek yogurt
- 1 tablespoon honey or maple syrup

Instructions:

1. Dice the mango into small pieces.
2. Blend the mango, carrot juice, Greek yogurt, and honey/maple syrup until the mixture is completely smooth.
3. If needed, strain the mixture to ensure it is free from lumps and fibers.

Nutritional Data:
Calories: 190 | Protein: 9g | Carbs: 35g | Fat: 2g | Fiber: 3g | Sugar: 30g

7. Soothing Pumpkin Pie Porridge

Preparation Time: 5 minutes | Cooking Time: 15 minutes

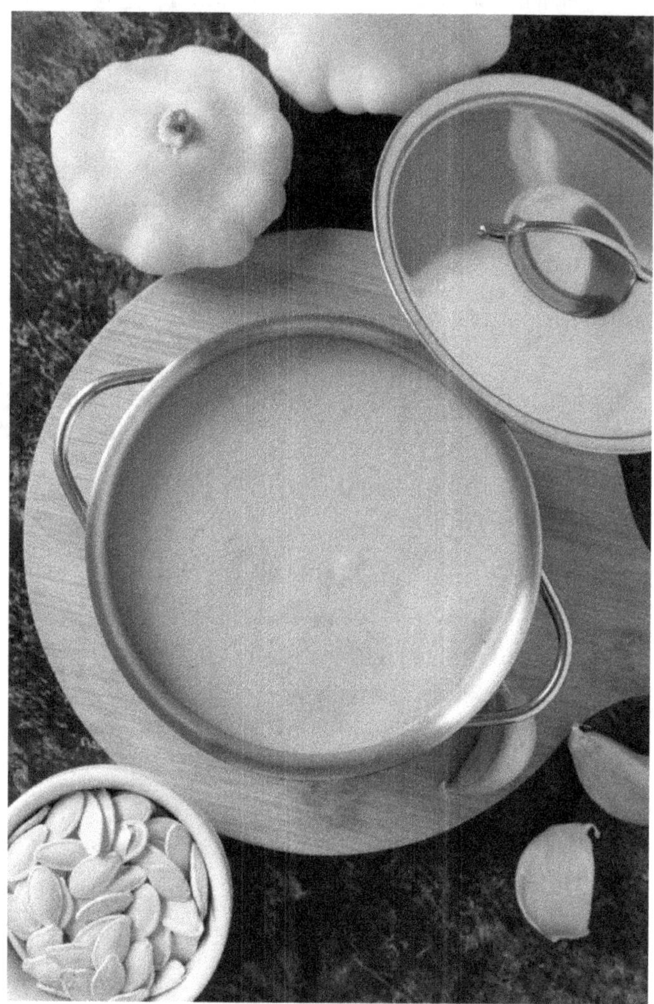

Ingredients:

- 1/2 cup finely ground rolled oats
- 1 cup water or milk (for cooking)
- 1/2 cup pumpkin puree (smooth, canned)
- 1/4 teaspoon ground cinnamon
- 1/4 teaspoon ground ginger
- 1 tablespoon maple syrup or honey (optional)
- Pinch of salt

Instructions:

1. In a saucepan, combine finely ground oats and water or milk. Stir continuously to prevent lumps.
2. Cook over medium heat until the mixture starts to thicken, about 5-7 minutes.
3. Reduce the heat to low. Add the pumpkin puree, cinnamon, ginger, maple syrup/honey (if using), and a pinch of salt. Mix well.
4. Continue to cook for another 5-8 minutes, stirring frequently, until the porridge reaches a very smooth, cohesive consistency.
5. Remove from heat and let it cool slightly. Ensure the porridge is lump-free and easy to swallow.

Nutritional Data:
Calories: 220 | Protein: 6g | Carbs: 45g | Fat: 2g | Fiber: 6g | Sugar: 12g

LEVEL 2 RECIPES

8.Soft Scrambled Eggs with Cheddar

Preparation Time: 5 minutes | Cooking Time: 5 minutes

Ingredients:

- 2 large eggs
- 1/4 cup shredded cheddar cheese
- 1 tablespoon milk or cream
- Salt and pepper to taste
- 1 teaspoon butter

Instructions:

1. In a bowl, whisk together the eggs, milk or cream, salt, and pepper.

2. Heat a non-stick skillet over low heat and melt the butter.
3. Pour the egg mixture into the skillet. Cook gently, stirring frequently, until the eggs are just set but still soft and creamy.
4. Remove from heat and gently fold in the shredded cheddar cheese until it's just melted and incorporated

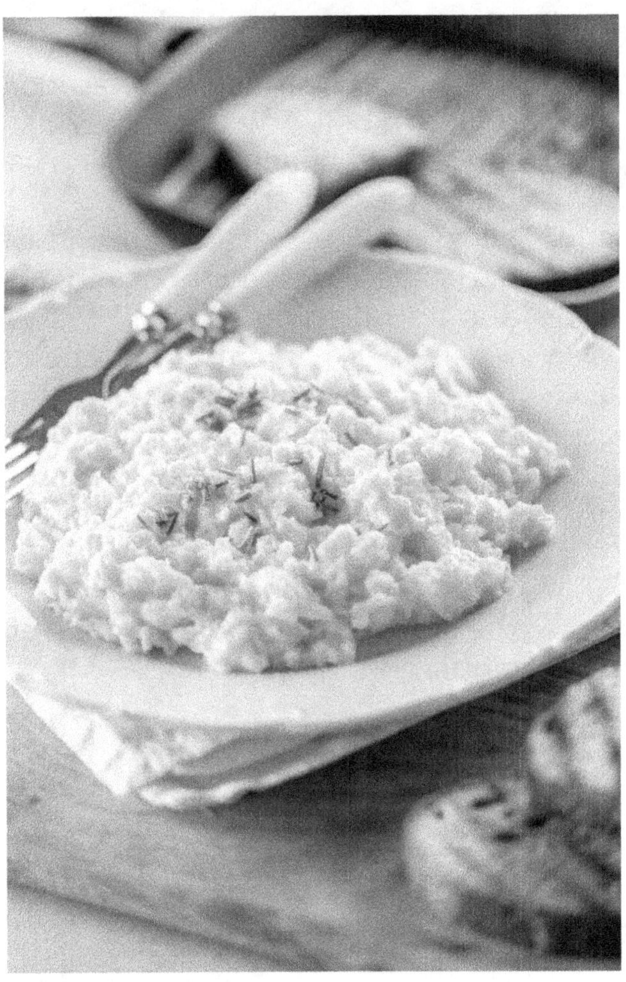

Nutritional Data:
Calories: 280 | Protein: 20g | Carbs: 2g | Fat: 22g | Fiber: 0g | Sugar: 1g

9.Tender Oatmeal with Stewed Fruit

Preparation Time: 5 minutes | Cooking Time: 15 minutes

Ingredients:

- 1/2 cup rolled oats
- 1 cup water or milk
- 1/2 cup mixed berries (fresh or frozen)
- 1 tablespoon honey or maple syrup
- A pinch of cinnamon

Instructions:

1. In a saucepan, bring the water or milk to a boil. Add the oats and reduce the heat to a simmer.
2. Cook the oats, stirring occasionally, until they are soft and have absorbed the liquid, about 10-15 minutes.
3. Meanwhile, in another pot, cook the berries with a splash of water and honey/maple syrup over medium heat until they form a soft, stewed consistency, about 5-10 minutes.
4. Serve the oatmeal topped with the stewed fruit and a sprinkle of cinnamon.

Nutritional Data:
Calories: 210 | Protein: 6g | Carbs: 42g | Fat: 3g | Fiber: 6g | Sugar: 15g

10.Moist Banana Bread Pudding

Preparation Time: 10 minutes | Cooking Time: 30 minutes

Ingredients:

- 1 ripe banana, mashed
- 1 slice of soft white bread, torn into small pieces
- 1/2 cup milk
- 1 egg, beaten
- 1 tablespoon sugar
- 1/4 teaspoon vanilla extract
- Pinch of cinnamon

Instructions:

1. Preheat the oven to 350°F (175°C).
2. In a bowl, combine the mashed banana, torn bread, milk, beaten egg, sugar, vanilla extract, and cinnamon. Mix until well combined.
3. Pour the mixture into a greased oven-safe dish.
4. Bake for about 30 minutes, or until the pudding is set and the top is golden brown.
5. Allow to cool slightly and serve warm.

Nutritional Data:
Calories: 330 | Protein: 11g | Carbs: 50g | Fat: 10g | Fiber: 3g | Sugar: 27g

11.Creamy Rice Pudding

Preparation Time: 5 minutes | Cooking Time: 30 minutes

Ingredients:

- 1/4 cup uncooked white rice
- 1 cup milk
- 1/4 cup heavy cream
- 2 tablespoons sugar
- 1/4 teaspoon vanilla extract
- Pinch of ground cinnamon

Instructions:

1. In a saucepan, combine the rice and milk. Bring to a boil, then reduce heat to low and simmer for 20 minutes, stirring occasionally.
2. Stir in the heavy cream, sugar, and vanilla extract. Continue to cook for another 10 minutes, until the rice is very soft and the mixture has thickened.

3. Remove from heat and sprinkle with a pinch of cinnamon.
4. Serve warm, ensuring the pudding is smooth and easily swallowable.

Nutritional Data:

Calories: 350 | Protein: 8g | Carbs: 50g | Fat: 14g | Fiber: 1g | Sugar: 25g

12.Fluffy Ricotta Pancakes

Preparation Time: 10 minutes | Cooking Time: 10 minutes

Ingredients:

- 1/2 cup ricotta cheese
- 1/4 cup all-purpose flour
- 1 egg
- 2 tablespoons milk
- 1 tablespoon sugar
- 1/2 teaspoon baking powder
- 1/4 teaspoon vanilla extract
- Butter for cooking

Instructions:

1. In a bowl, mix the ricotta cheese, egg, milk, and vanilla extract.
2. In another bowl, combine the flour, sugar, and baking powder.
3. Gradually add the dry ingredients to the wet ingredients, stirring until just combined.
4. Heat a non-stick skillet over medium heat and add a small amount of butter.
5. Pour small amounts of the batter onto the skillet. Cook until bubbles form on the surface, then flip and cook until golden brown.
6. Serve warm. If needed, the pancakes can be lightly pureed or mashed to ensure a soft, moist texture.

Nutritional Data:

Calories: 400 | Protein: 20g | Carbs: 35g | Fat: 20g | Fiber: 1g | Sugar: 12g

13.Soft Poached Pears in Cinnamon Syrup

Preparation Time: 10 minutes | Cooking Time: 20 minutes

Ingredients:

- 1 ripe pear, peeled and cored
- 1 cup water
- 1/4 cup sugar
- 1 cinnamon stick
- 1/4 teaspoon lemon juice

Instructions:

1. In a saucepan, combine water, sugar, cinnamon sticks, and lemon juice. Bring to a simmer.
2. Add the pear to the saucepan and simmer gently until the pear is soft about 15-20 minutes.
3. Remove the pear and let it cool slightly.
4. If necessary, mash or lightly puree the pear to achieve a soft, smooth consistency.
5. Serve the pear warm with some of the cinnamon syrup drizzled over it.

Nutritional Data:

Calories: 230 | Protein: 1g | Carbs: 60g | Fat: 0g | Fiber: 5g | Sugar: 50g

14.Cottage Cheese with Soft Peach Compote

Preparation Time: 5 minutes | Cooking Time: 10 minutes

Ingredients:

- 1/2 cup cottage cheese
- 1 ripe peach, peeled and diced
- 1 tablespoon water
- 1 tablespoon honey or sugar
- 1/4 teaspoon cinnamon

Instructions:

1. In a small saucepan, combine the diced peach, water, honey or sugar, and cinnamon. Cook over medium heat, stirring occasionally, until the peaches are very soft and the mixture resembles a compote, about 10 minutes.
2. Let the peach compote cool slightly. If needed, mash it gently to ensure a soft texture.
3. Serve the warm peach compote over the cottage cheese.

Nutritional Data: Calories: 180 | Protein: 14g | Carbs: 25g | Fat: 4g | Fiber: 2g | Sugar: 22g

LEVEL 3 RECIPES

15.Moist French Toast

Preparation Time: 10 minutes | Cooking Time: 5 minutes

Ingredients:

- 2 slices of soft, white bread
- 1 egg
- 1/4 cup whole milk
- 1/2 tsp vanilla extract
- Pinch of ground cinnamon
- 1 tbsp unsalted butter
- Maple syrup or fruit puree for topping (optional)

Instructions:

1. In a shallow bowl, beat the egg with milk, vanilla extract, and cinnamon until well combined.
2. Dip each slice of bread into the egg mixture, allowing it to soak for a few seconds on each side.
3. Melt butter in a non-stick skillet over medium heat.
4. Place the soaked bread slices in the skillet and cook for about 2 minutes on each side, until golden brown and cooked through.
5. Serve warm with a drizzle of maple syrup or fruit puree if desired.

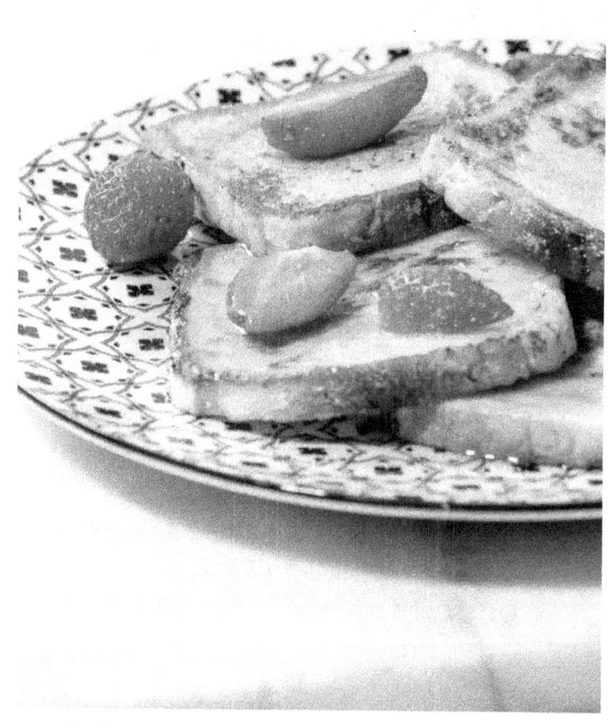

Nutritional Data:

Calories: 350 | Protein: 12g | Carbohydrates: 45g | Fat: 15g | Fiber: 2g | Sugar: 10g

16. Soft Baked Omelet

Preparation Time: 5 minutes | Cooking Time: 15 minutes

Ingredients:

- 2 large eggs
- 2 tbsp whole milk
- 1/4 cup shredded cheddar cheese
- 1/4 cup cooked, chopped spinach
- Salt and pepper to taste
- 1 tbsp unsalted butter

Instructions:

1. Preheat the oven to 350°F (175°C).
2. In a bowl, whisk together eggs, milk, salt, and pepper.
3. Stir in the cheese and spinach.
4. Grease a small oven-safe dish with butter.
5. Pour the egg mixture into the dish.
6. Bake for 15 minutes, or until the omelet is set and slightly golden on top.
7. Let it cool for a few minutes before serving.

Nutritional Data:

Calories: 300 | Protein: 20g | Carbohydrates: 4g | Fat: 23g | Fiber: 1g | Sugar: 2g

17. Creamy Banana Oatmeal with Pureed Berries

Preparation Time: 15 minutes | Cooking Time: 20 minutes

Ingredients:

- 1/2 cup rolled oats (for smooth texture)
- 1 ripe banana (for natural sweetness and smooth texture)
- 1 cup almond milk or any preferred non-dairy milk (for creaminess and easier swallowing)
- 1/2 tsp ground cinnamon (for flavor)
- 1/4 cup mixed berries (blueberries, strawberries, raspberries), pureed
- Optional: A drizzle of honey or maple syrup for added sweetness
- Optional: A pinch of salt (to enhance flavors)

Instructions:

1. In a small pot, combine the rolled oats and almond milk. Bring to a simmer over medium heat.
2. Cook for about 5-7 minutes, stirring frequently, until the oatmeal is soft and has a creamy consistency.
3. Mash the ripe banana and stir it into the oatmeal along with the ground cinnamon. Cook for another 2-3 minutes until everything is well combined and the banana is fully incorporated into the oatmeal.
4. While the oatmeal is cooking, puree the mixed berries using a blender or a food processor until smooth. If needed, you can add a little water or juice to achieve a moderately thick, smooth consistency.
5. Once the oatmeal is cooked to a smooth consistency, remove it from heat. Let it cool down a bit to a safe temperature.
6. Serve the oatmeal in a bowl, topped with the berry puree. Drizzle with a little honey or maple syrup if desired.

Nutritional Data:
Calories: 300 per muffin | Protein: 6g |
Carbohydrates: 50g | Fat: 5g | Fiber: 5g |
Sugar: 15g

18.Creamy Polenta with Cheese

Preparation Time: 5 minutes | Cooking Time: 25 minutes

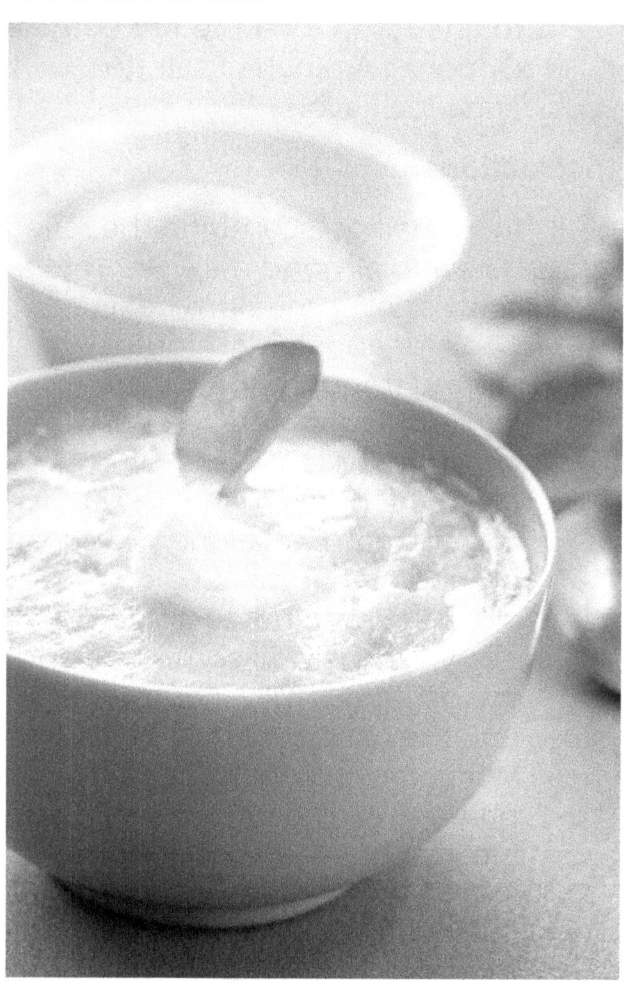

Ingredients:

- 1/4 cup polenta (cornmeal)
- 1 cup water
- 1/4 cup grated Parmesan cheese
- 1 tbsp unsalted butter
- Salt to taste

Instructions:

1. In a medium saucepan, bring water to a boil.
2. Gradually whisk in the polenta and reduce heat to low.
3. Cook, stirring frequently, until the polenta thickens and is creamy, about 20-25 minutes.
4. Remove from heat and stir in the butter and Parmesan cheese until well combined.
5. Season with salt to taste.
6. Serve warm, ensuring the texture is smooth and suitable for swallowing.

Nutritional Data:
Calories: 300 | Protein: 10g |
Carbohydrates: 33g | Fat: 15g | Fiber: 2g
| Sugar: 1g

19.Soft Pancakes with Maple Syrup

Preparation Time: 10 minutes | Cooking Time: 10 minutes

Ingredients:

- 1 cup all-purpose flour
- 1 tbsp sugar
- 1 tsp baking powder
- 1/2 tsp baking soda
- Pinch of salt
- 3/4 cup buttermilk
- 1 large egg
- 2 tbsp unsalted butter, melted
- Maple syrup for serving

Instructions:

1. In a large bowl, whisk together flour, sugar, baking powder, baking soda, and salt.
2. In another bowl, mix buttermilk, egg, and melted butter.
3. Pour the wet ingredients into the dry ingredients and stir until just combined.

4. Heat a non-stick skillet over medium heat and lightly grease with butter.
5. Pour 1/4 cup of batter for each pancake and cook until bubbles form on the surface, then flip and cook until golden brown.
6. Serve warm with maple syrup.

Nutritional Data:
Calories: 600 | Protein: 15g | Carbohydrates: 85g | Fat: 23g | Fiber: 2g | Sugar: 30g

20.Avocado Toast on Soft Bread

Preparation Time: 5 minutes | Cooking Time: 2 minutes

Ingredients:

- 1 slice of soft, white bread
- 1/2 ripe avocado
- Salt to taste
- A squeeze of lemon juice (optional)

Instructions:

1. Toast the bread slice until it is just lightly toasted, maintaining a soft texture.
2. Mash the avocado with a fork and season with salt and lemon juice.
3. Spread the mashed avocado evenly over the toast.
4. Cut into small, manageable pieces for easy swallowing.

Nutritional Data:
Calories: 230 | Protein: 4g | Carbohydrates: 30g | Fat: 12g | Fiber: 5g | Sugar: 3g

21.Cinnamon-Apple Soft Baked Bars

Preparation Time: 15 minutes | Cooking Time: 25 minutes

Ingredients:

- 1 cup all-purpose flour
- 1/2 cup rolled oats
- 1/2 cup brown sugar
- 1 tsp baking powder
- 1/2 tsp ground cinnamon
- Pinch of salt
- 1/2 cup unsweetened applesauce
- 1/4 cup unsalted butter, melted
- 1 egg
- 1/2 tsp vanilla extract

Instructions:

1. Preheat the oven to 350°F (175°C) and line an 8x8 inch baking dish with parchment paper.
2. In a large bowl, mix flour, oats, brown sugar, baking powder, cinnamon, and salt.
3. In another bowl, combine applesauce, melted butter, egg, and vanilla extract.
4. Add the wet ingredients to the dry ingredients and mix until just combined.
5. Pour the batter into the prepared baking dish, spreading evenly.
6. Bake for 25 minutes or until a toothpick inserted into the center comes out clean.
7. Let cool completely in the dish, then cut into bars.

Nutritional Data:
Calories: 200 per bar | Protein: 3g | Carbohydrates: 35g | Fat: 6g | Fiber: 2g | Sugar: 18g

LEVEL 4 RECIPES

22.Soft Scrambled Eggs with Herbs

Preparation Time: 5 minutes | Cooking Time: 5 minutes

Ingredients:

- 2 large eggs
- 1 tbsp whole milk
- 1 tsp unsalted butter
- 1 tbsp chopped fresh herbs (such as parsley, chives, or dill)
- Salt and pepper to taste

Instructions:

1. In a bowl, whisk together the eggs, milk, salt, and pepper.
2. Melt butter in a non-stick skillet over low heat.
3. Pour the egg mixture into the skillet. Let it sit without stirring for 1 minute.
4. Gently stir the eggs with a spatula, folding them over in large, soft curds.
5. Remove from heat when the eggs are set but still moist and slightly runny.
6. Stir in the chopped herbs and serve immediately.

Nutritional Data:
Calories: 200 | Protein: 14g | Carbohydrates: 1g | Fat: 15g | Fiber: 0g | Sugar: 1g

23.Creamy Greek Yogurt with Honey and Soft Fruits

Preparation Time: 5 minutes | Cooking Time: 0 minutes

Ingredients:

- 1 cup Greek yogurt, plain
- 1 tbsp honey
- 1/2 cup soft fruits, such as banana slices or ripe peach

Instructions:

1. In a serving bowl, combine the Greek yogurt with honey.
2. Top with soft fruits, ensuring they are ripe and easy to swallow.
3. Gently mix or serve with the fruit on top.

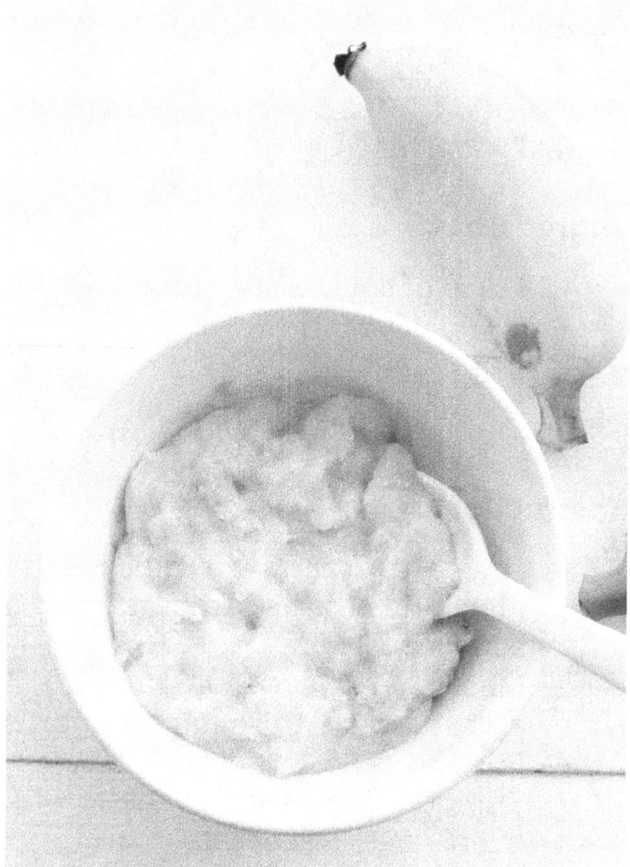

Nutritional Data:
Calories: 250 | Protein: 15g | Carbohydrates: 35g | Fat: 7g | Fiber: 2g | Sugar: 30g

24.Tender Vegetable Frittata

Preparation Time: 10 minutes | Cooking Time: 15 minutes

Ingredients:

- 2 large eggs
- 1/4 cup whole milk
- 1/2 cup cooked vegetables (like zucchini, bell pepper, and spinach), finely chopped
- 1/4 cup shredded cheddar cheese
- 1 tbsp unsalted butter
- Salt and pepper to taste

Instructions:

1. Preheat the oven to 375°F (190°C).
2. In a bowl, whisk together eggs, milk, salt, and pepper.
3. Stir in the cooked vegetables and cheese.
4. Heat butter in an oven-proof skillet over medium heat.
5. Pour the egg mixture into the skillet, stirring gently to distribute the vegetables.
6. Cook without stirring until the edges begin to set, about 3-4 minutes.
7. Transfer the skillet to the oven and bake for 10-12 minutes until the frittata is set.
8. Let it cool slightly and cut into small, manageable pieces.

Nutritional Data:

Calories: 350 | Protein: 20g | Carbohydrates: 5g | Fat: 28g | Fiber: 1g | Sugar: 3g

25.Cottage Cheese and Soft Peach Bowl

Preparation Time: 5 minutes | Cooking Time: 0 minutes

Ingredients:

- 1/2 cup cottage cheese
- 1 ripe peach, peeled and diced
- A drizzle of honey (optional)

Instructions:

1. In a serving bowl, place the cottage cheese.
2. Top with soft, diced peach.
3. Drizzle with honey if desired.
4. Gently mix or serve as is.

Nutritional Data:

Calories: 200 | Protein: 14g | Carbohydrates: 20g | Fat: 6g | Fiber: 2g | Sugar: 18g

26.Moist Banana-Walnut Bread

Preparation Time: 15 mins | Cooking Time: 1 hour

Ingredients:

- 2 ripe bananas, mashed
- 1 cup all-purpose flour
- 3/4 cup sugar
- 2 eggs, beaten
- 1/2 cup walnuts, finely chopped

Instructions:

1. Preheat oven to 350°F (175°C). Grease a loaf pan.
2. In a mixing bowl, combine mashed bananas with sugar and beaten eggs.
3. Stir in flour and finely chopped walnuts until just combined.
4. Pour the batter into the prepared loaf pan.
5. Bake for 1 hour or until a toothpick inserted into the center comes out clean.
6. Allow the bread to cool before serving to ensure a safe temperature.

Nutritional Data:

Calories: 330 | Carbohydrates: 53g | Protein: 6g | Fat: 12g | Sodium: 200mg | Fiber: 2g

27.Soft Whole Grain Waffles

Preparation Time: 10 mins | Cooking Time: 5 mins per waffle

Ingredients:

- 1 cup whole grain waffle mix
- 3/4 cup milk
- 2 eggs
- Soft toppings: yogurt or fruit compote

Instructions:

1. Heat a waffle iron according to the manufacturer's instructions.
2. In a bowl, whisk together the waffle mix, milk, and eggs until smooth.
3. Pour enough batter into the waffle iron to just cover the waffle grid.
4. Cook for about 5 minutes or until the waffle is golden brown and slightly crisp.
5. Serve warm with a dollop of yogurt or a spoonful of fruit compote on top.

Nutritional Data:
Calories: 290 | Carbohydrates: 38g | Protein: 11g | Fat: 10g | Sodium: 430mg | Fiber: 5g

28. Avocado and Soft-Boiled Egg Toast

Preparation Time: 10 minutes | Cooking Time: 6 minutes

Ingredients:

- 1 ripe avocado
- 1 large egg
- 1 slice of soft whole-grain bread

Instructions:

1. Soft-boil the egg: Place the egg in a saucepan and cover with water. Bring to a boil, then reduce heat and simmer for 6 minutes. Remove the egg from the saucepan and place it in cold water to stop the cooking process.
2. Peel the egg and set it aside.
3. Cut the avocado in half, remove the pit, and scoop out the flesh into a bowl.
4. Mash the avocado with a fork until it reaches a smooth, creamy consistency.
5. Toast the bread until it is just warm and soft, not crispy.
6. Spread the mashed avocado evenly over the toast.
7. Slice the soft-boiled egg and place it on top of the avocado.
8. Serve immediately.

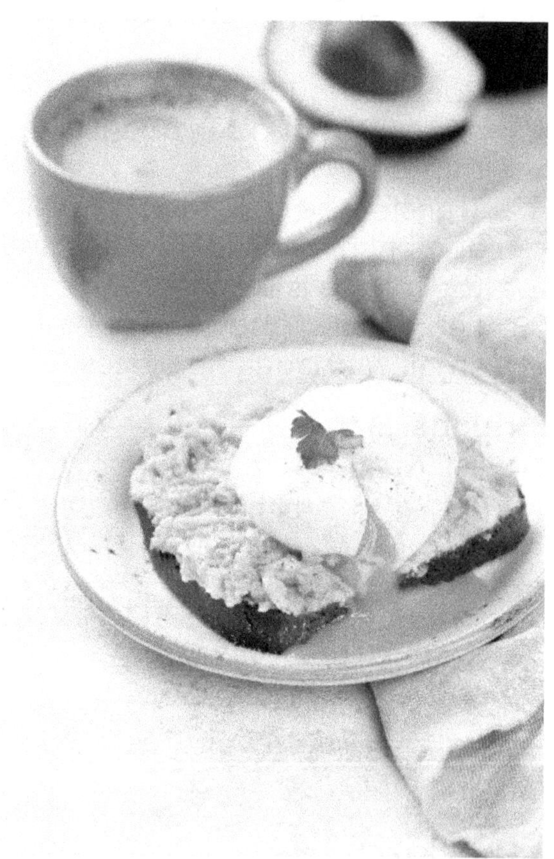

Nutritional Data:
Calories: 300 | Protein: 10g | Carbohydrates: 19g | Fat: 20g | Fiber: 5g | Sugar: 2g

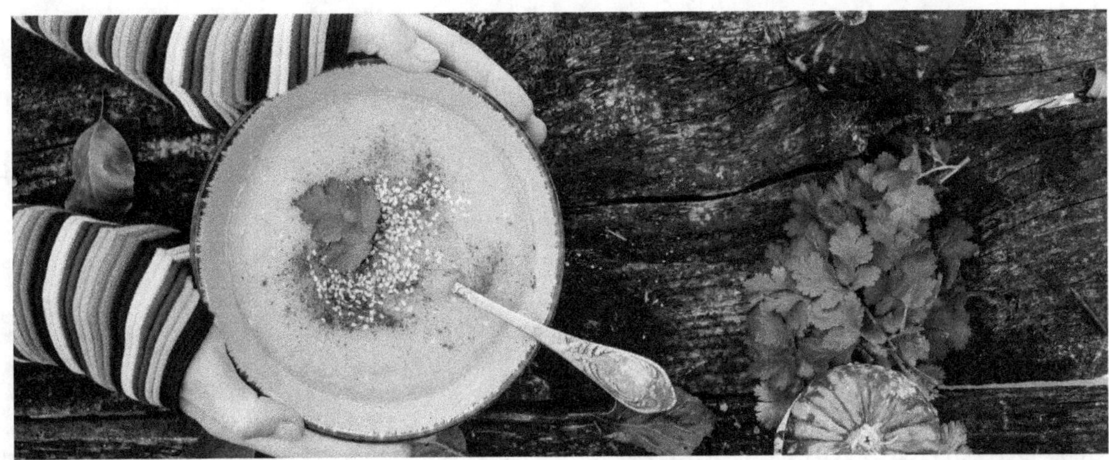

Nourishing Soups and Stews

This section is a heartwarming collection of recipes designed to provide warmth, comfort, and nutrition, all while adhering to the specific needs of those with dysphagia. Soups and stews are not only versatile and easy to adapt to various texture requirements, but they also offer an excellent way to hydrate and nourish in a single, delightful dish.

In this chapter, we celebrate the simplicity and versatility of soups and stews, offering recipes that range from rich, creamy blends to hearty, softly chunked meals. Each recipe is crafted with care, ensuring it can be modified to suit different levels of dysphagia, providing safe and enjoyable eating experiences for all.

For the Pureed Diet (Level 1), we have a selection of silky smooth soups, velvety and full of flavor. Think of classic favorites like cream of tomato or pumpkin soup, each pureed to perfection, ensuring a safe, smooth texture without compromising on taste.

At the Soft and Well-Cooked level (Level 2), the recipes evolve to include soups with soft, well-cooked ingredients that are easy to chew and swallow, such as tender vegetable minestrone or soft lentil stew.

Moving to **Advanced Textures (Level 3),** our recipes introduce slightly more texture while still focusing on softness and ease of swallowing. This section features dishes like chunky potato soup and hearty barley stew, all prepared to be gentle on the swallow.

For those on the **Regular Diet with Modifications (Level 4),** the soups and stews become more robust, incorporating a wider range of ingredients while still being mindful of size, texture, and ease of eating. Recipes like beef stew and chicken noodle soup are adjusted to ensure they are safe and enjoyable.

Each recipe in this chapter is more than just a meal; it's a soothing embrace in a bowl, designed to bring pleasure and nutrition in every spoonful. With these soups and stews, you'll find that maintaining a dysphagia diet doesn't have to mean missing out on the flavors and textures that make food enjoyable.

LEVEL 1 RECIPES

29. Creamy Butternut Squash Soup

Preparation Time: 15 mins | Cooking Time: 30 mins

Ingredients:

- 1 cup butternut squash, peeled and cubed
- 2 cups vegetable broth
- 1/4 cup chopped onion
- 1/4 tsp ground nutmeg
- 1/4 tsp ground ginger

Instructions:

1. In a large pot, combine the butternut squash, vegetable broth, and onion. Bring to a boil.
2. Reduce heat and simmer until the squash is very tender about 25 minutes.
3. Remove from heat and let it cool slightly.
4. Add nutmeg and ginger.
5. Using a blender or immersion blender, puree the soup until smooth.
6. Return the pureed soup to the pot and heat through. If the soup is too thick, add a little extra broth to reach the desired consistency.
7. Serve warm.

Nutritional Data:

Calories: 90 | Carbohydrates: 22g | Protein: 2g | Fat: 0.2g | Sodium: 480mg | Fiber: 3g

30. Silky Carrot and Ginger Soup

Preparation Time: 10 mins | Cooking Time: 20 mins

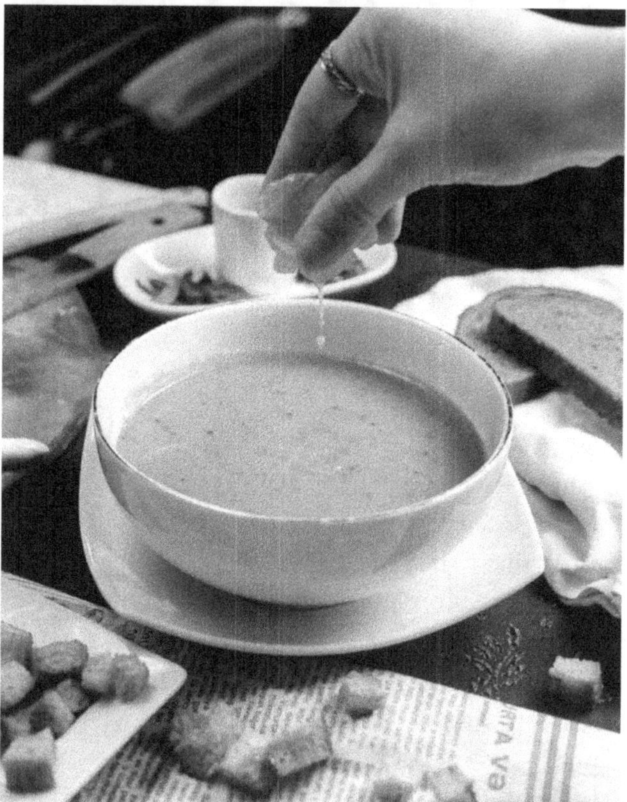

Ingredients:

- 1 cup carrots, peeled and sliced
- 1 tbsp fresh ginger, grated
- 1/4 cup chopped onion
- 2 cups vegetable broth
- 1/4 cup cream

Instructions:

1. In a large pot, add carrots, ginger, onion, and vegetable broth.
2. Bring to a boil, then lower the heat and simmer until carrots are very tender about 15-20 minutes.
3. Let the mixture cool slightly.
4. Puree the mixture in a blender until completely smooth.
5. Return the pureed soup to the pot, stir in the cream, and heat through.

6. If necessary, adjust the consistency with additional broth or water.
7. Serve warm, ensuring the soup is at a comfortable temperature.

Nutritional Data:
Calories: 120 | Carbohydrates: 13g | Protein: 2g | Fat: 7g | Sodium: 410mg | Fiber: 3g

31. Velvety Potato and Leek Soup

Preparation Time: 15 mins | Cooking Time: 25 mins

Ingredients:

- 1 cup potatoes, peeled and chopped
- 1/2 cup leeks, cleaned and sliced
- 2 cups chicken or vegetable broth
- 1/4 cup cream

Instructions:

1. In a pot, combine potatoes, leeks, and broth. Bring to a boil.
2. Reduce heat and simmer until potatoes are very tender about 20 minutes.
3. Let the mixture cool slightly.
4. Puree the soup in a blender until completely smooth.
5. Return the pureed soup to the pot, stir in the cream, and heat through.
6. Adjust consistency with additional broth if needed.
7. Serve warm, ensuring it's at a comfortable temperature for eating.

Nutritional Data:
Calories: 150 | Carbohydrates: 21g | Protein: 3g | Fat: 7g | Sodium: 410mg | Fiber: 2g

32. Smooth Tomato Basil Soup

Preparation Time: 10 mins | Cooking Time: 30 mins

Ingredients:

- 1 cup ripe tomatoes, chopped
- 1/4 cup fresh basil leaves
- 1/4 cup onion, chopped
- 1 clove garlic, minced
- 2 cups vegetable broth

Instructions:

1. In a pot, sauté onions and garlic until soft.
2. Add chopped tomatoes and vegetable broth, and bring to a boil.
3. Reduce heat and simmer for 25 minutes.
4. Add basil leaves in the last 5 minutes of cooking.
5. Let the soup cool slightly.
6. Puree the soup in a blender until smooth.
7. Reheat the soup, adjusting consistency with additional broth if necessary.
8. Serve warm.

Nutritional Data:
Calories: 70 | Carbohydrates: 16g | Protein: 2g | Fat: 0.5g | Sodium: 480mg | Fiber: 3g

33. Pureed Pea and Mint Soup

Preparation Time: 10 mins | Cooking Time: 20 mins

Ingredients:

- 1 cup green peas (fresh or frozen)
- 2 tbsp fresh mint leaves
- 1/4 cup onion, chopped
- 2 cups vegetable broth
- 1/4 cup cream

Instructions:

1. In a saucepan, sauté onions until translucent.
2. Add green peas and vegetable broth, and bring to a boil.
3. Simmer for 15 minutes or until the peas are very soft.
4. Add mint leaves in the last few minutes of cooking.
5. Let the mixture cool slightly.
6. Puree the soup in a blender until completely smooth.
7. Stir in cream and gently reheat the soup.
8. Serve warm, ensuring it's at a comfortable temperature.

Nutritional Data:

Calories: 120 | Carbohydrates: 15g | Protein: 4g | Fat: 6g | Sodium: 410mg | Fiber: 4g

34. Creamy Broccoli Soup

Preparation Time: 15 mins | Cooking Time: 25 mins

Ingredients:

- 1 cup broccoli florets
- 1 clove garlic, minced
- 1/4 cup onion, chopped
- 2 cups chicken or vegetable broth
- 1/4 cup cream

Instructions:

1. In a saucepan, sauté garlic and onion until soft.
2. Add broccoli and broth, and bring to a boil.
3. Simmer until broccoli is very tender, about 20 minutes.
4. Let the soup cool slightly.
5. Blend the soup in a blender until smooth.
6. Return the soup to the saucepan, stir in cream, and heat through.
7. Adjust the consistency with additional broth if needed.
8. Serve the soup warm.

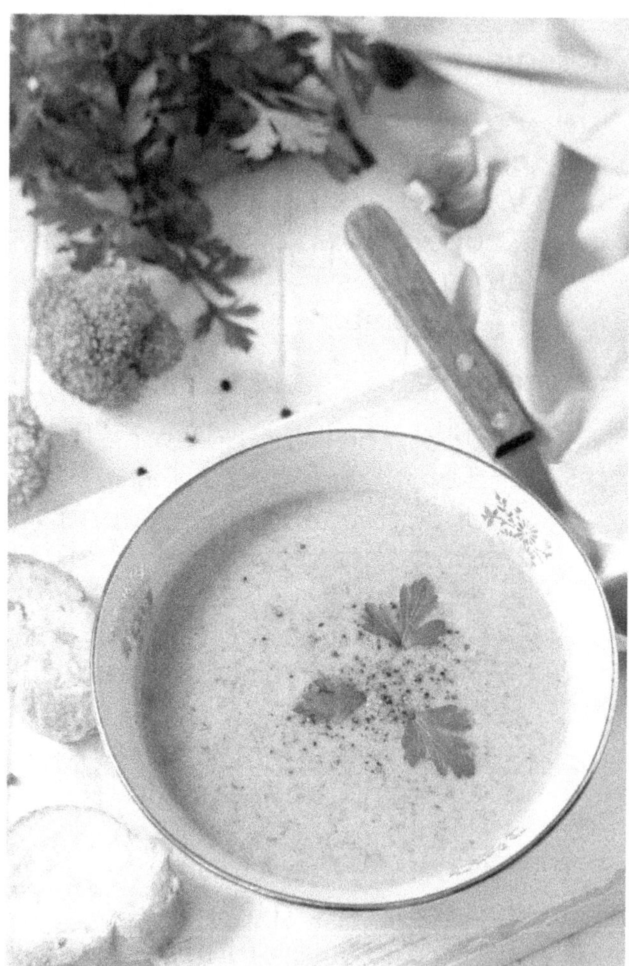

Nutritional Data:

Calories: 130 | Carbohydrates: 10g | Protein: 5g | Fat: 8g | Sodium: 470mg | Fiber: 3g

35. Pumpkin and Apple Soup

Preparation Time: 15 mins | Cooking Time: 30 mins

Ingredients:

- 1 cup pumpkin puree
- 1 medium apple, peeled and chopped
- 1/4 cup onion, chopped
- 2 cups vegetable broth
- 1/2 tsp cinnamon

Instructions:

1. In a large pot, sauté onions until they become translucent.
2. Add chopped apples and cook until they begin to soften.
3. Stir in the pumpkin puree, vegetable broth, and cinnamon.
4. Bring the mixture to a boil, then reduce heat and simmer for about 20-25 minutes, until all ingredients are very soft.
5. Allow the soup to cool slightly.
6. Using a blender, puree the soup until it reaches a smooth consistency.
7. Reheat the soup gently, adding more broth if needed to adjust the thickness.
8. Ensure the soup is at a comfortable temperature before serving.

Nutritional Data:

Calories: 80 | Carbohydrates: 19g | Protein: 2g | Fat: 0.5g | Sodium: 480mg | Fiber: 4g

LEVEL2 RECIPES

36. Soft Lentil and Vegetable Soup

Preparation Time: 15 mins | Cooking Time: 45 mins

Ingredients:

- 1/2 cup lentils, rinsed
- 1/2 cup carrots, chopped
- 1/2 cup celery, chopped
- 1/4 cup onion, chopped
- 3 cups vegetable broth

Instructions:

1. In a large pot, sauté onions, carrots, and celery until softened.
2. Add lentils and vegetable broth. Bring to a boil.
3. Reduce heat to a simmer. Cover and cook until lentils and vegetables are very tender, about 40 minutes.
4. Allow the soup to cool slightly.
5. Using a blender, puree the soup until it reaches a soft, manageable consistency.
6. Reheat the soup gently. If it's too thick, add more broth to achieve the desired texture.
7. Serve warm, ensuring it's at a comfortable temperature.

Nutritional Data:

Calories: 150 | Carbohydrates: 28g | Protein: 9g | Fat: 0.5g | Sodium: 410mg | Fiber: 8g

37. Tender Chicken and Rice Soup

Preparation Time: 20 mins | Cooking Time: 35 mins

Ingredients:

- 1 cup chicken breast, cooked and chopped
- 1/2 cup rice
- 2 cups chicken broth
- 1/2 cup carrots, chopped
- 1/2 cup celery, chopped

Instructions:

1. In a large pot, bring the chicken broth to a boil.
2. Add the rice, carrots, and celery. Reduce heat to a simmer.
3. Cook until the vegetables and rice are very soft, about 20 minutes.
4. Add the cooked chicken to the pot and continue to simmer until the chicken is heated through.
5. Allow the soup to cool slightly.
6. Carefully blend the soup to a soft, manageable consistency, suitable for Level 2 dysphagia.
7. Reheat the soup if necessary, adjusting the texture with additional broth if needed.
8. Serve warm.

Nutritional Data:

Calories: 190 | Carbohydrates: 23g | Protein: 18g | Fat: 3g | Sodium: 480mg | Fiber: 2g

38. Creamy Cauliflower and Cheese Soup

Preparation Time: 10 mins | Cooking Time: 25 mins

Ingredients:

- 1 cup cauliflower, chopped
- 1/2 cup mild cheese, grated
- 1 cup milk
- 1 cup vegetable broth
- A pinch of nutmeg

Instructions:

1. In a pot, combine cauliflower and vegetable broth. Bring to a boil.
2. Reduce heat and simmer until cauliflower is very soft about 20 minutes.
3. Stir in milk, cheese, and nutmeg until the cheese is melted and the mixture is well combined.
4. Let the mixture cool slightly.
5. Using a blender, puree the soup until it reaches a soft, manageable consistency for Dysphagia Level 2.
6. Reheat the soup gently, adding more milk or broth if needed to adjust the thickness.
7. Serve the soup warm, ensuring it's at a comfortable temperature.

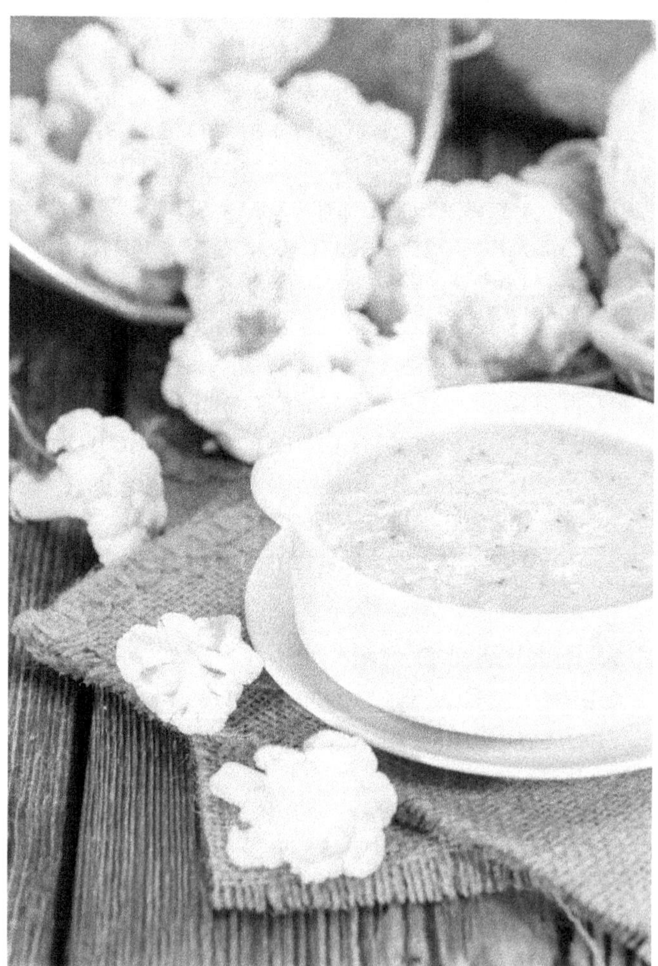

Nutritional Data:
Calories: 180 | Carbohydrates: 13g |
Protein: 10g | Fat: 10g | Sodium: 500mg
| Fiber: 2g

39. Soft Split Pea Soup with Ham

Preparation Time: 15 mins | Cooking Time: 1 hour 30 mins

Ingredients:

- 1/2 cup split peas
- 1/2 cup ham, cooked and diced
- 1/4 cup onion, chopped
- 1/2 cup carrots, chopped
- 3 cups chicken or vegetable broth

Instructions:

1. In a large pot, combine split peas, ham, onions, carrots, and broth. Bring to a boil.
2. Reduce heat to a simmer, cover, and cook until peas and vegetables are very soft, about 1 hour and 20 minutes.
3. Allow the soup to cool slightly.
4. Puree the soup in a blender, in batches if necessary, until smooth but still suitable for Dysphagia Level 2, with a bit of texture.
5. Reheat the soup gently, thinning with additional broth if necessary.
6. Serve warm, checking for temperature and consistency.

Nutritional Data:
Calories: 210 | Carbohydrates: 25g |
Protein: 15g | Fat: 5g | Sodium: 670mg |
Fiber: 6g

40. Gentle Beef and Potato Stew

Preparation Time: 20 mins | Cooking Time: 2 hours

Ingredients:

- 1 cup beef stew meat, cut into small pieces
- 1 cup potatoes, peeled and chopped
- 1/2 cup carrots, peeled and chopped
- 2 cups beef broth
- 1 tsp dried mixed herbs

Instructions:

1. In a large pot, brown the beef stew meat over medium heat.
2. Add potatoes, carrots, beef broth, and mixed herbs to the pot.
3. Bring to a boil, then reduce the heat to low and let it simmer, covered, until the beef is very tender, about 1 hour and 45 minutes.
4. Allow the stew to cool slightly.
5. Blend the stew using a blender or immersion blender until it reaches a soft consistency suitable for Dysphagia Level 2.
6. Reheat the stew gently, adding more broth if needed to adjust the thickness.
7. Serve warm, ensuring the stew is at a comfortable temperature.

Nutritional Data:
Calories: 220 | Carbohydrates: 20g |
Protein: 25g | Fat: 6g | Sodium: 550mg |
Fiber: 3g

41. Soft Barley and Mushroom Soup

Preparation Time: 15 mins | Cooking Time: 40 mins

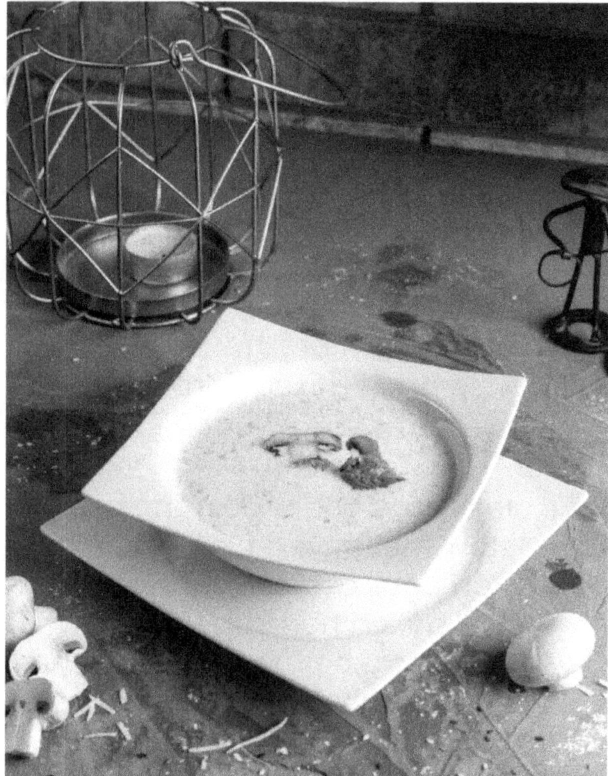

Ingredients:

- 1/2 cup barley
- 1 cup mushrooms, cleaned and sliced
- 1/4 cup onion, chopped
- 3 cups vegetable or chicken broth
- 1/2 tsp dried thyme

Instructions:

1. In a pot, sauté onions and mushrooms until they are soft.
2. Add barley, broth, and thyme to the pot.
3. Bring to a boil, then reduce heat to a simmer. Cover and cook until the barley is very soft, about 30 minutes.
4. Allow the soup to cool slightly.
5. Carefully blend the soup to a soft consistency suitable for Dysphagia Level 2, ensuring no large chunks are remaining.
6. Reheat the soup gently, adding more broth if needed to adjust the thickness.
7. Serve warm, checking to ensure the soup is at a safe temperature to eat

Nutritional Data:
Calories: 180 | Carbohydrates: 35g | Protein: 6g | Fat: 1g | Sodium: 480mg | Fiber: 8g

42. Smooth Pumpkin Bisque

Preparation Time: 10 mins | Cooking Time: 30 mins

Ingredients:

- 1 cup pumpkin puree (canned or fresh)
- 1/4 cup onion, finely chopped
- 1 tsp fresh ginger, grated
- 2 cups vegetable broth
- 1/4 cup cream

Instructions:

1. In a large pot, sauté the onion and ginger until the onion is translucent.
2. Add the pumpkin puree and vegetable broth, stirring to combine.
3. Bring the mixture to a boil, then reduce heat to a simmer and cook for about 20 minutes, allowing the flavors to meld.
4. Remove from heat and let cool slightly.
5. Using an immersion blender or standard blender, puree the soup until it is completely smooth and

at a suitable consistency for Dysphagia Level 2.

6. Return the bisque to the pot and stir in the cream, warming gently over low heat.
7. Once the bisque is heated through, check the consistency, adding a little more broth if necessary.
8. Serve warm, ensuring it's not too hot for safe consumption.

Nutritional Data:
Calories: 200 | Carbohydrates: 18g | Protein: 2g | Fat: 14g | Sodium: 410mg | Fiber: 5g

LEVEL3 RECIPES

43. Chunky Potato and Leek Soup

Preparation Time: 15 minutes | Cooking Time: 30 minutes

Ingredients:

- 1 large potato, peeled and diced
- 1 leek, white and light green parts only, finely chopped
- 1 cup chicken or vegetable broth
- 1/2 cup cream
- 1 tbsp unsalted butter
- Salt and pepper to taste

Instructions:

1. In a saucepan, melt butter over medium heat. Add chopped leeks and cook until soft, about 5 minutes.
2. Add diced potatoes and broth. Bring to a boil, then reduce heat and simmer until the potatoes are very tender about 20 minutes.

3. Stir in the cream and heat through without boiling—season with salt and pepper.
4. For a smoother consistency, blend the soup partially or fully with an immersion blender.
5. Serve warm, ensuring the chunks are soft and easy to swallow.

Nutritional Data:
Calories: 350 | Protein: 4g | Carbohydrates: 40g | Fat: 20g | Fiber: 3g | Sugar: 4g

44. Tender Chicken Noodle Soup

Preparation Time: 15 minutes | Cooking Time: 25 minutes

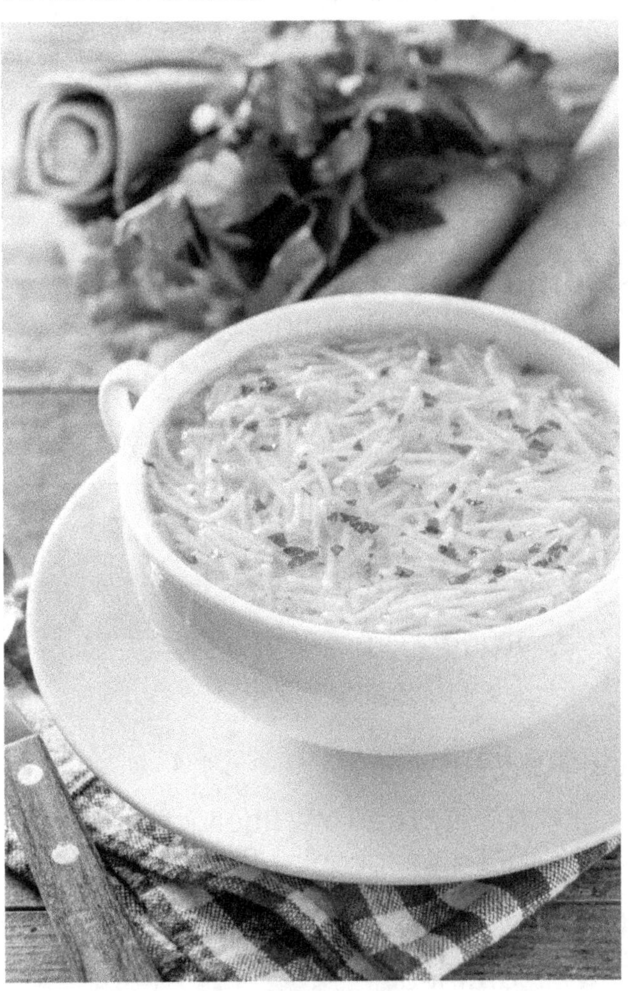

Ingredients:

- 4 oz chicken breast, cooked and shredded
- 1/2 cup thin egg noodles
- 1 small carrot, peeled and finely chopped
- 1 stick of celery, finely chopped
- 2 cups chicken broth

Instructions:

1. In a pot, bring chicken broth to a boil.
2. Add carrots and celery, and simmer until they are soft about 10 minutes.
3. Add the cooked chicken and noodles to the pot. Cook until the noodles are soft, about 5-10 minutes.
4. If needed, further shred the chicken to ensure it is very tender and easy to swallow.
5. Adjust seasoning with salt and pepper.
6. Serve warm, with a focus on a soft, cohesive texture.

Nutritional Data:

Calories: 300 | Protein: 25g | Carbohydrates: 30g | Fat: 7g | Fiber: 2g | Sugar: 3g

45. Hearty Minestrone with Soft Vegetables

Preparation Time: 20 minutes | Cooking Time: 30 minutes

Ingredients:

- 1/2 cup carrots, finely chopped
- 1/2 cup zucchini, finely chopped
- 1/2 cup canned beans (such as cannellini or kidney), rinsed and drained
- 1/2 cup small pasta shapes
- 1 cup canned tomatoes, chopped
- 2 cups vegetable broth
- 1 tbsp olive oil
- Salt and pepper to taste

Instructions:

1. In a large pot, heat olive oil over medium heat. Add carrots and cook until they start to soften about 5 minutes.
2. Add zucchini and cook for another 5 minutes.
3. Pour in the vegetable broth and bring to a simmer.
4. Add the canned tomatoes, beans, and pasta. Simmer until the pasta and vegetables are very soft, about 20 minutes.
5. Season with salt and pepper to taste.
6. For a smoother consistency, blend the soup partially or fully with an immersion blender.
7. Serve warm, ensuring all ingredients are soft and easy to swallow.

Nutritional Data:

Calories: 300 | Protein: 10g | Carbohydrates: 50g | Fat: 7g | Fiber: 10g | Sugar: 8g

46. Creamy Fish Chowder

Preparation Time: 15 minutes | Cooking Time: 25 minutes

Ingredients:

- 4 oz white fish (such as cod or haddock), cut into small pieces
- 1 small potato, peeled and diced
- 1/2 cup onion, finely chopped
- 1 cup fish or vegetable broth
- 1/2 cup milk or cream
- 1 tbsp unsalted butter

- Salt and pepper to taste
- Fresh parsley, finely chopped (optional)

Instructions:

1. In a saucepan, melt butter over medium heat. Add onions and cook until translucent.
2. Add the diced potatoes and broth. Bring to a boil, then reduce heat and simmer until potatoes are tender about 10-15 minutes.
3. Add the fish to the saucepan. Cook until the fish is easily flaked with a fork, about 5-10 minutes.
4. Reduce the heat to low. Stir in milk or cream, and gently heat through without boiling—season with salt and pepper.
5. If desired, use an immersion blender to blend the chowder to a smooth consistency.
6. Garnish with parsley if using, and serve warm.

Nutritional Data:
Calories: 300 | Protein: 18g | Carbohydrates: 25g | Fat: 15g | Fiber: 2g | Sugar: 5g

47. Soft Beef and Barley Stew

Preparation Time: 20 minutes | Cooking Time: 2 hours

Ingredients:

- 4 oz beef stew meat, cut into small pieces
- 1/4 cup barley
- 1/2 cup carrots, diced
- 2 cups beef broth
- 1 tsp dried herbs (such as thyme or rosemary)
- 1 tbsp olive oil
- Salt and pepper to taste

Instructions:

1. In a pot, heat olive oil over medium heat. Brown the beef pieces, then remove and set aside.
2. In the same pot, add carrots and cook until slightly softened.
3. Return the beef to the pot and add barley, beef broth, and herbs.
4. Bring to a boil, then reduce heat to low and simmer, covered, for about 2 hours, or until the beef and barley are very tender.
5. Season with salt and pepper to taste.
6. Before serving, ensure the beef and barley are soft enough to be easily swallowed. If necessary, blend the stew to a suitable consistency.

Nutritional Data:
Calories: 450 | Protein: 30g | Carbohydrates: 35g | Fat: 20g | Fiber: 6g | Sugar: 3g

48. Butternut Squash and Carrot Soup

Preparation Time: 15 minutes | Cooking Time: 30 minutes

Ingredients:

- 1 cup butternut squash, peeled and diced
- 1/2 cup carrots, diced
- 1/4 cup onion, finely chopped
- 2 cups vegetable broth
- 1/4 cup cream
- 1 tbsp olive oil
- Salt and pepper to taste

Instructions:

1. In a pot, heat olive oil over medium heat. Add onion and cook until translucent.
2. Add butternut squash and carrots. Cook for about 5 minutes.
3. Pour in the vegetable broth and bring to a boil. Reduce heat and simmer until the vegetables are very soft about 25 minutes.
4. Stir in the cream and warm through.
5. Blend the soup until smooth, ensuring any pieces are small and soft.
6. Season with salt and pepper to taste.
7. Serve warm, with a focus on a smooth, creamy texture.

Nutritional Data:

Calories: 300 | Protein: 3g | Carbohydrates: 40g | Fat: 15g | Fiber: 6g | Sugar: 10g

49. Mildly Spiced Lentil Stew

Preparation Time: 15 minutes | Cooking Time: 45 minutes

Ingredients:

- 1/2 cup lentils, rinsed
- 1/2 cup carrots, finely chopped
- 1/2 cup celery, finely chopped
- 1 cup canned tomatoes, chopped
- 2 cups vegetable or chicken broth
- 1 tsp mild spice mix (such as cumin, coriander, and paprika)
- 1 tbsp olive oil
- Salt and pepper to taste

Instructions:

1. In a pot, heat olive oil over medium heat. Add carrots and celery, cooking until they start to soften, about 5 minutes.
2. Stir in the spice mix, cooking for another minute to release the flavors.
3. Add lentils, canned tomatoes, and broth. Bring to a boil.
4. Reduce heat to low and simmer, covered, for about 40 minutes or until lentils and vegetables are very tender.
5. Season with salt and pepper to taste.
6. If needed, blend the stew for a smoother texture, ensuring it's suitable for easy swallowing.
7. Serve warm, focusing on a soft, cohesive consistency.

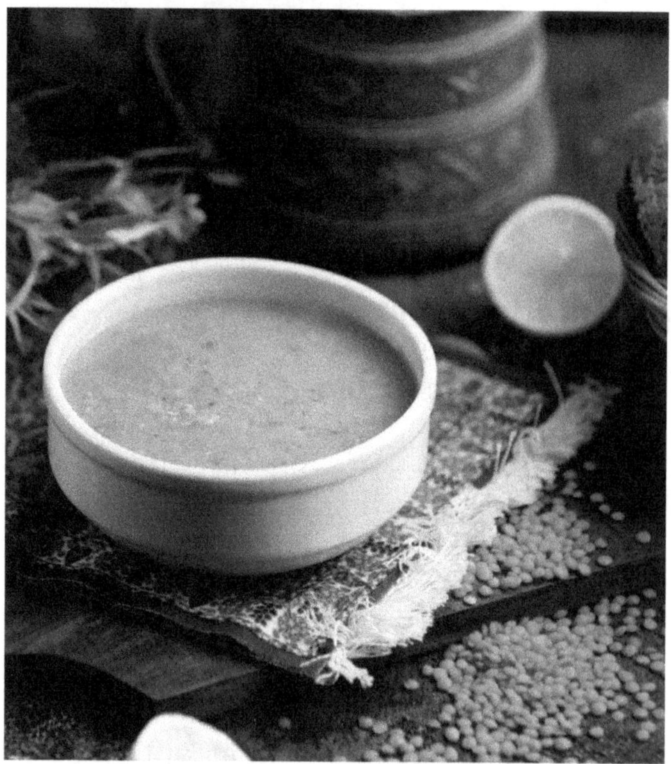

Nutritional Data:

Calories: 350 | Protein: 18g | Carbohydrates: 60g | Fat: 7g | Fiber: 15g | Sugar: 10g

LEVEL4 RECIPES

50. Hearty Vegetable Beef Stew

Preparation Time: 20 minutes | Cooking Time: 1 hour 30 minutes

Ingredients:

- 4 oz beef stew meat, cut into small pieces
- 1/2 cup carrots, diced
- 1/2 cup potatoes, diced
- 1/4 cup peas
- 2 cups beef broth
- 1 tsp dried herbs (such as thyme or rosemary)
- 1 tbsp olive oil
- Salt and pepper to taste

Instructions:

1. In a pot, heat olive oil over medium heat. Brown the beef pieces, then remove and set aside.
2. Add carrots and potatoes to the pot, cooking until they start to soften, about 10 minutes.
3. Return the beef to the pot. Add peas, beef broth, and herbs.
4. Bring to a boil, then reduce heat to low and simmer, covered, for about 1 hour 30 minutes, until the beef and vegetables are very tender.
5. Season with salt and pepper to taste.
6. Before serving, check the tenderness of the beef and vegetables. Blend the stew if needed to ensure a soft, cohesive consistency suitable for Level 4 Dysphagia.

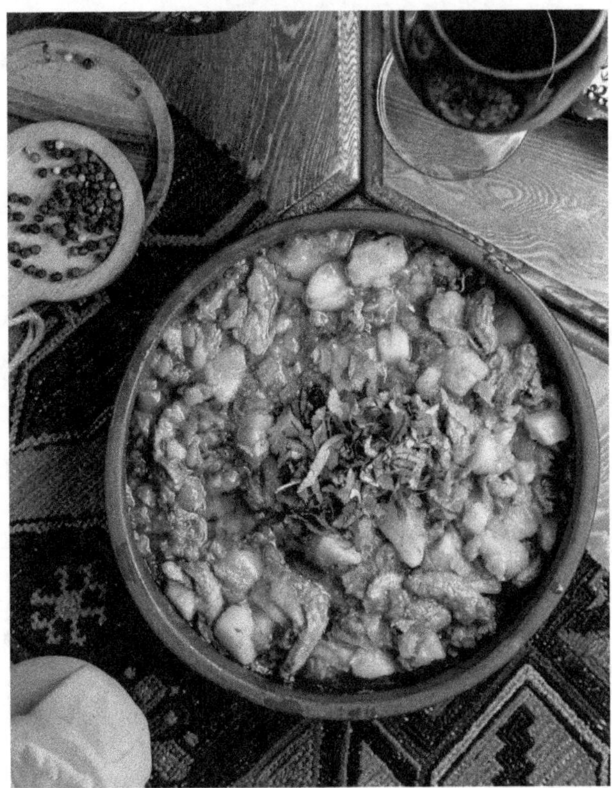

Nutritional Data:
Calories: 500 | Protein: 35g | Carbohydrates: 40g | Fat: 22g | Fiber: 5g | Sugar: 5g

51. Creamy Chicken and Wild Rice Soup

Preparation Time: 15 minutes | Cooking Time: 45 minutes

Ingredients:

- 4 oz chicken breast, cooked and shredded
- 1/4 cup wild rice
- 1/2 cup carrots, diced
- 1/2 cup celery, diced
- 2 cups chicken broth
- 1/2 cup cream
- Salt and pepper to taste

Instructions:

1. In a pot, bring chicken broth to a boil. Add wild rice and simmer for about 30 minutes.

2. Add carrots and celery, cooking until they are tender, about 15 minutes.
3. Add the cooked, shredded chicken and cream, heating through gently without boiling.
4. Season with salt and pepper to taste.
5. Before serving, ensure the chicken and vegetables are tender enough to be easily swallowed. Blend partially or fully if needed for a suitable texture.

Nutritional Data:
Calories: 400 | Protein: 25g | Carbohydrates: 30g | Fat: 20g | Fiber: 3g | Sugar: 5g

52. Tuscan White Bean and Kale Soup

Preparation Time: 15 minutes | Cooking Time: 30 minutes

Ingredients:

- 1/2 cup white beans, canned or pre-cooked
- 1 cup kale, finely chopped
- 1 cup canned tomatoes, chopped
- 2 cups vegetable broth
- 1 tsp Italian herbs
- 1 tbsp olive oil
- Salt and pepper to taste

Instructions:

1. In a pot, heat olive oil over medium heat. Add the Italian herbs and cook for a minute to release their flavor.
2. Add the white beans, canned tomatoes, and vegetable broth. Bring to a boil.
3. Reduce heat and simmer for about 20 minutes.

4. Add the kale and cook until it's tender, about 10 minutes.
5. Season with salt and pepper to taste.
6. Before serving, blend the soup to ensure a smooth, consistent texture that's suitable for Dysphagia Level 4.
7. Serve warm.

Nutritional Data:
Calories: 250 | Protein: 12g | Carbohydrates: 40g | Fat: 7g | Fiber: 10g | Sugar: 6g

53. Tomato Basil Bisque with Soft Mozzarella

Preparation Time: 10 minutes | Cooking Time: 20 minutes

Ingredients:

- 2 cups ripe tomatoes, chopped
- 1/4 cup fresh basil, chopped
- 1/4 cup mozzarella cheese, finely diced
- 1/2 onion, finely chopped
- 2 cups vegetable or chicken broth
- 1 tbsp olive oil
- Salt and pepper to taste

Instructions:

1. In a pot, heat olive oil over medium heat. Add the onion and cook until translucent.
2. Add the tomatoes and cook for about 5 minutes, until they start to soften.
3. Pour in the broth and bring to a boil. Reduce heat and simmer for 15 minutes.
4. Add the basil and simmer for an additional 5 minutes.
5. Blend the soup until smooth.

6. Stir in the mozzarella cheese until it melts into the soup.
7. Season with salt and pepper to taste.
8. Serve warm, ensuring the soup is smooth and the cheese is fully melted.

Nutritional Data:
Calories: 220 | Protein: 8g | Carbohydrates: 18g | Fat: 14g | Fiber: 4g | Sugar: 10g

54. Mushroom and Barley Soup

Preparation Time: 10 minutes | Cooking Time: 40 minutes

Ingredients:

- 1/2 cup barley
- 1 cup mushrooms, finely chopped
- 1/2 onion, finely chopped
- 2 cups beef or vegetable broth
- 1 tsp dried thyme
- 1 tbsp olive oil
- Salt and pepper to taste

Instructions:

1. In a pot, heat olive oil over medium heat. Add onions and cook until translucent.
2. Add mushrooms and thyme, cooking for about 5 minutes until the mushrooms are soft.
3. Pour in the broth and add the barley. Bring to a boil.
4. Reduce heat to low and simmer, covered, for about 35 minutes, or until the barley is tender.
5. Season with salt and pepper to taste.
6. Before serving, blend the soup partially or completely, depending on the desired

consistency, ensuring it's suitable for Dysphagia Level 4.
7. Serve warm.

Nutritional Data:
Calories: 260 | Protein: 8g | Carbohydrates: 45g | Fat: 7g | Fiber: 10g | Sugar: 4g

55. Sweet Potato and Corn Chowder

Preparation Time: 15 minutes | Cooking Time: 30 minutes

Ingredients:

- 1 large sweet potato, peeled and diced
- 1/2 cup corn kernels
- 1/2 onion, finely chopped
- 2 cups vegetable or chicken broth
- 1/2 cup milk or cream
- 1 tbsp olive oil
- Salt and pepper to taste

Instructions:

1. In a pot, heat olive oil over medium heat. Add the onion and cook until translucent.
2. Add sweet potato and corn. Cook for about 5 minutes.
3. Pour in the broth and bring to a boil. Reduce heat and simmer until the sweet potatoes are tender about 20 minutes.
4. Stir in the milk or cream and warm through.
5. Blend the chowder to a smooth consistency, ensuring it's suitable for Dysphagia Level 4.
6. Season with salt and pepper to taste.
7. Serve warm.

Nutritional Data:
Calories: 300 | Protein: 5g | Carbohydrates: 50g | Fat: 10g | Fiber: 5g | Sugar: 10g

56. Savory Pumpkin and Ginger Soup

Preparation Time: 10 minutes | Cooking Time: 20 minutes

Ingredients:

- 1 cup pumpkin puree
- 1/2 tsp fresh ginger, finely grated
- 1 cup vegetable broth
- 1/4 cup cream
- A pinch of cinnamon
- Salt and pepper to taste

Instructions:

1. In a pot, combine the pumpkin puree, ginger, and vegetable broth. Stir well.
2. Bring the mixture to a boil over medium heat, then reduce to a simmer.
3. Add a pinch of cinnamon and simmer for about 15 minutes, allowing the flavors to meld together.
4. Stir in the cream and heat through, ensuring not to boil.
5. Season with salt and pepper to taste.
6. For a smoother consistency, blend the soup until it reaches a uniform texture, suitable for Dysphagia Level 4.
7. Serve warm, enjoying the comforting blend of pumpkin and ginger.

Nutritional Data:
Calories: 200 | Protein: 2g | Carbohydrates: 25g | Fat: 10g | Fiber: 6g | Sugar: 8g

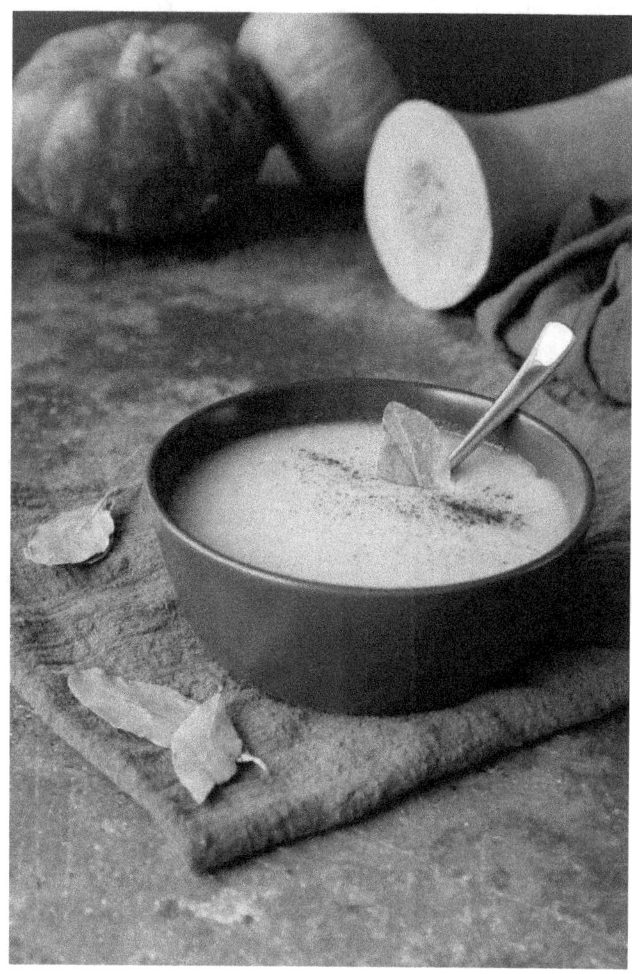

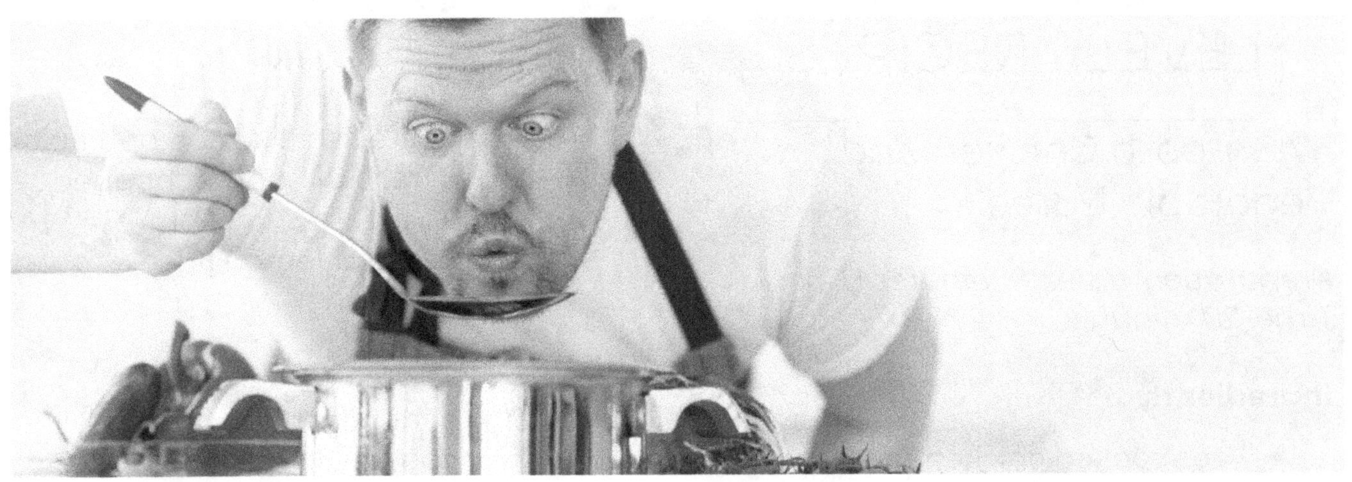

Main Courses

This section is dedicated to bringing variety, flavor, and nutrition to the centerpiece of your meal, all while catering to the specific needs of those with dysphagia. We understand the importance of having a satisfying main dish that is not only safe to swallow but also appealing and fulfilling.

In these pages, you will find a diverse array of main course recipes, each thoughtfully designed to suit different dysphagia diet levels. From comforting casseroles to tender, flavorful meats, and savory vegetarian options, there's something to please every palate. These dishes ensure that the main event at your dining table is both a culinary delight and a safe, nutritious option for those with swallowing difficulties.

For individuals on a Pureed Diet (Level 1), the focus is on finely pureed, smooth, and cohesive dishes that are easy on the swallow yet rich in flavor. Imagine pureed chicken with gravy or a smooth vegetable casserole, both packed with taste and nutrition.

As we move to the Soft and Well-Cooked level (Level 2), the recipes offer a bit more texture. Soft, tender meatloaf or moist, flaky fish prepared in a way that's easy to chew and swallow, providing both comfort and variety.

Advancing to the Advanced Textures (Level 3), the main courses begin to resemble more typical meals, yet remain mindful of texture and ease of swallowing. Dishes like soft baked chicken or tender beef stroganoff make their appearance, satisfying the desire for more traditional fare.

For those on the **Regular Diet with Modifications (Level 4),** the recipes broaden to include a full range of ingredients, thoughtfully prepared to ensure safety. Here, you'll find dishes like modified stir-fries or soft, yet flavorful, pasta dishes, catering to a more standard diet while still considering dysphagia needs.

Each recipe in this section is a testament to the fact that a dysphagia diet can be diverse and delicious. We strive to make mealtimes an occasion to look forward to, with main dishes that are as nutritious as they are appetizing.

LEVEL 1 RECIPES

57.Smooth Chicken and Vegetable Puree

Preparation Time: 10 minutes | Cooking Time: 20 minutes

Ingredients:

- 4 oz cooked chicken breast
- 1/2 cup carrots, peeled and chopped
- 1/2 cup peas
- 1 cup chicken broth
- Salt to taste

Instructions:

1. Cook the carrots in boiling water until very tender, about 10 minutes. Add peas in the last 3 minutes of cooking.
2. In a blender, combine the cooked chicken, carrots, peas, and chicken broth.
3. Blend until the mixture reaches a very smooth consistency.
4. Add salt to taste and blend again to incorporate.
5. If needed, adjust the thickness by adding more broth to reach the desired consistency for Dysphagia Level 1.
6. Serve warm, ensuring the puree is smooth and uniform.

Nutritional Data:
Calories: 220 | Protein: 28g | Carbohydrates: 15g | Fat: 4g | Fiber: 4g | Sugar: 5g

58. Creamy Pureed Fish with Dill

Preparation Time: 10 minutes | Cooking Time: 15 minutes

Ingredients:

- 4 oz white fish (like cod or tilapia)
- 1 tbsp fresh dill, finely chopped
- 1/4 cup cream
- A squeeze of lemon juice
- Salt to taste

Instructions:

1. Steam or poach the fish until it is fully cooked and flakes easily.
2. In a blender, combine the cooked fish, dill, cream, and a squeeze of lemon juice.
3. Blend until completely smooth.
4. Add salt to taste and blend again to incorporate.
5. Adjust consistency with additional cream or water, aiming for a smooth, uniform puree suitable for Dysphagia Level 1.
6. Serve warm, ensuring the puree is fine and consistent.

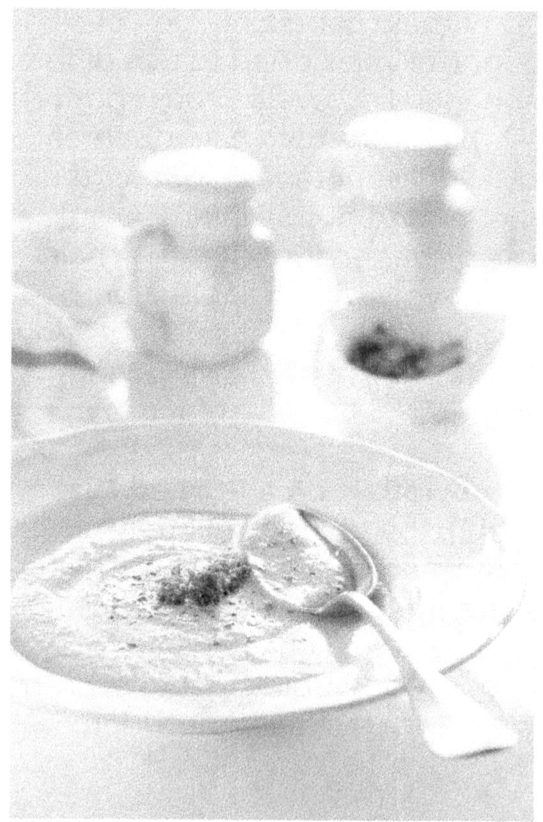

Nutritional Data:
Calories: 180 | Protein: 22g |
Carbohydrates: 2g | Fat: 10g | Fiber: 0g |
Sugar: 1g

59. Velvety Beef and Potato Puree

*Preparation Time: 20 minutes |
Cooking Time: 2 hours*

Ingredients:

- 4 oz beef stew meat
- 1 large potato, peeled and diced
- 1 cup beef broth
- 1 tsp dried rosemary
- Salt to taste

Instructions:

1. In a pot, combine the beef, potatoes, beef broth, and rosemary.
2. Bring to a boil, then reduce heat to low and simmer for about 2 hours, or until the beef and potatoes are extremely tender.
3. Once cooked, transfer the beef, potatoes, and a bit of the cooking liquid to a blender.
4. Blend until the mixture is completely smooth and velvety.
5. Add salt to taste and adjust the consistency by adding more cooking liquid if necessary.
6. Serve warm, ensuring the puree is fine and uniform in texture.

Nutritional Data:
Calories: 300 | Protein: 28g |
Carbohydrates: 35g | Fat: 6g | Fiber: 4g |
Sugar: 2g

60. Silken Tofu and Spinach Blend

Preparation Time: 5 minutes | Cooking Time: 10 minutes

Ingredients:

- 1/2 cup silken tofu
- 1 cup spinach, steamed
- 1 small garlic clove, finely minced
- 1 tbsp olive oil
- Salt to taste

Instructions:

1. Steam the spinach until it is very soft, about 5-10 minutes.
2. In a blender, combine the steamed spinach, silken tofu, minced garlic, and olive oil.
3. Blend until the mixture is smooth and creamy.
4. Add salt to taste and blend again to incorporate.
5. Adjust the consistency by adding a little water or additional olive oil if needed.
6. Serve warm, ensuring the blend is smooth and homogeneous.

Nutritional Data:
Calories: 150 | Protein: 10g |
Carbohydrates: 6g | Fat: 10g | Fiber: 2g |
Sugar: 1g

61. Pureed Turkey with Gravy

Preparation Time: 10 minutes | Cooking Time: 20 minutes

Ingredients:

- 4 oz cooked turkey breast
- 1/2 cup turkey or chicken broth
- Salt and pepper to taste

Instructions:

1. Cut the cooked turkey breast into small pieces.
2. In a blender, combine the turkey pieces and broth.
3. Blend until the mixture reaches a very smooth consistency.
4. Season with salt and pepper, and blend again to incorporate.
5. If necessary, adjust the thickness by adding more broth to achieve a smooth puree suitable for Dysphagia Level 1.
6. Serve warm, ensuring the puree is uniform and easy to swallow.

Nutritional Data:
Calories: 150 | Protein: 25g | Carbohydrates: 0g | Fat: 3g | Fiber: 0g | Sugar: 0g

62. Savory Lentil and Carrot Puree

Preparation Time: 10 minutes | Cooking Time: 30 minutes

Ingredients:

- 1/2 cup cooked lentils
- 1/2 cup carrots, peeled and chopped
- 1 cup vegetable broth
- Mild spices (such as cumin or coriander), to taste
- Salt to taste

Instructions:

1. Cook the carrots in boiling water until very tender, about 20 minutes.
2. In a blender, combine the cooked lentils, carrots, and vegetable broth.
3. Add mild spices and salt.
4. Blend until the mixture is completely smooth and uniform.

5. Adjust the consistency by adding more broth if necessary, aiming for a smooth puree suitable for Dysphagia Level 1.
6. Serve warm, ensuring the puree is soft and cohesive.

Nutritional Data:
Calories: 200 | Protein: 12g | Carbohydrates: 35g | Fat: 1g | Fiber: 15g | Sugar: 5g

63. Butternut Squash and Apple Puree

Preparation Time: 10 minutes | Cooking Time: 30 minutes

Ingredients:

- 1 cup butternut squash, peeled and cubed
- 1 medium apple, peeled and chopped
- A pinch of cinnamon
- 1 cup vegetable broth

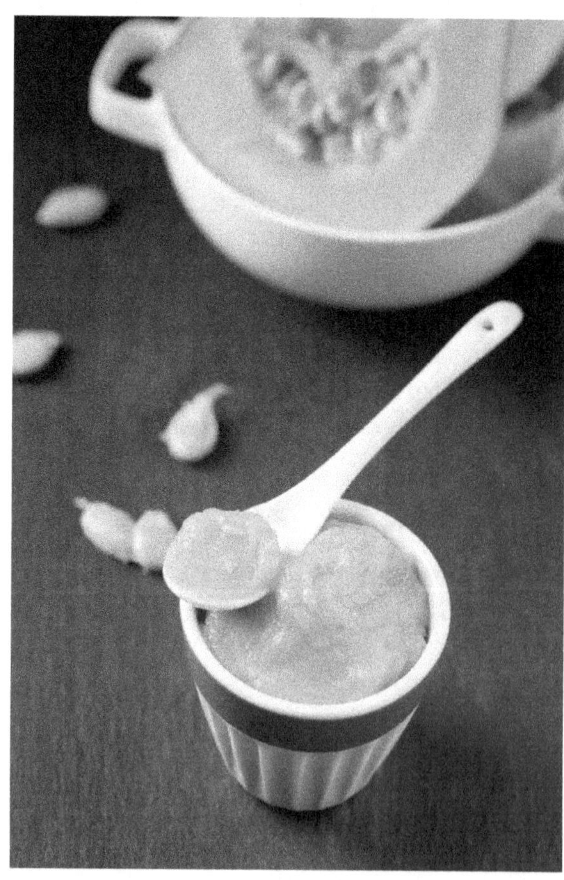

Instructions:

1. In a pot, add the butternut squash and apple. Cover with vegetable broth.
2. Bring to a boil, then reduce heat and simmer until both the squash and apple are very tender about 25-30 minutes.
3. Add a pinch of cinnamon to the mixture.
4. Transfer the contents to a blender, including the cooking liquid.
5. Blend until the mixture is completely smooth and uniform.
6. Adjust the consistency by adding more broth if necessary, to achieve a smooth puree suitable for Dysphagia Level 1.
7. Serve warm, ensuring the puree is silky and easy to swallow.

Nutritional Data:

Calories: 150 | Protein: 2g | Carbohydrates: 35g | Fat: 0.5g | Fiber: 6g | Sugar: 18g

LEVEL2 RECIPES

64. Soft Chicken and Rice Casserole

Preparation Time: 10 minutes | Cooking Time: 30 minutes

Ingredients:

- 4 oz cooked chicken breast, finely shredded
- 1/2 cup soft-cooked rice
- 1/2 cup cream of chicken soup
- Salt and pepper to taste

Instructions:

1. Preheat the oven to 350°F (175°C).
2. In a bowl, mix the finely shredded chicken, cooked rice, and cream of chicken soup until well combined.
3. Season with salt and pepper.
4. Transfer the mixture to a baking dish and spread evenly.
5. Bake in the preheated oven for 30 minutes, or until heated through and the top is slightly golden.
6. Before serving, gently mash the casserole to ensure the consistency is suitable for Dysphagia Level 2.

Nutritional Data:

Calories: 350 | Protein: 30g | Carbohydrates: 40g | Fat: 10g | Fiber: 1g | Sugar: 2g

65. Tender Meatloaf with Gravy

Preparation Time: 15 minutes | Cooking Time: 1 hour

Ingredients:

- 4 oz ground beef or turkey
- 1/4 cup breadcrumbs
- 1/4 cup milk
- 1 egg, beaten
- Seasoning to taste (such as salt, pepper, and a mild herb blend)
- 1/2 cup smooth gravy

Instructions:

1. Preheat the oven to 350°F (175°C).
2. In a bowl, combine the ground meat, breadcrumbs, milk, egg, and seasoning. Mix until well combined.
3. Transfer the mixture to a loaf pan and shape it into a loaf.
4. Bake for 1 hour, or until the meatloaf is cooked through.

5. Remove from the oven and let it cool slightly.
6. Finely mince the meatloaf or blend it to ensure a very soft, cohesive texture.
7. Serve with smooth gravy, ensuring the meatloaf and gravy are easy to swallow for Dysphagia Level 2.

Nutritional Data:
Calories: 400 | Protein: 25g | Carbohydrates: 20g | Fat: 22g | Fiber: 1g | Sugar: 3g

66. Moist Salmon Patties

Preparation Time: 15 minutes | Cooking Time: 10 minutes

Ingredients:

- 4 oz cooked salmon, finely flaked
- 1/4 cup soft breadcrumbs
- 1 egg, beaten
- 1 tbsp chopped herbs (such as dill or parsley)
- Salt and pepper to taste
- 1 tbsp olive oil for pan-frying

Instructions:

1. In a bowl, combine the finely flaked salmon, breadcrumbs, beaten egg, herbs, salt, and pepper. Mix until well combined.
2. Form the mixture into small patties.
3. Heat olive oil in a pan over medium heat.
4. Gently pan-fry the salmon patties for about 5 minutes on each side, until they are cooked through and have a soft texture.
5. Before serving, ensure that the patties are moist and easy to chew for Dysphagia Level 2.

Nutritional Data:
Calories: 300 | Protein: 25g | Carbohydrates: 15g | Fat: 15g | Fiber: 1g | Sugar: 2g

67. Creamy Mashed Potato and Cheese Bake

Preparation Time: 15 minutes | Cooking Time: 20 minutes

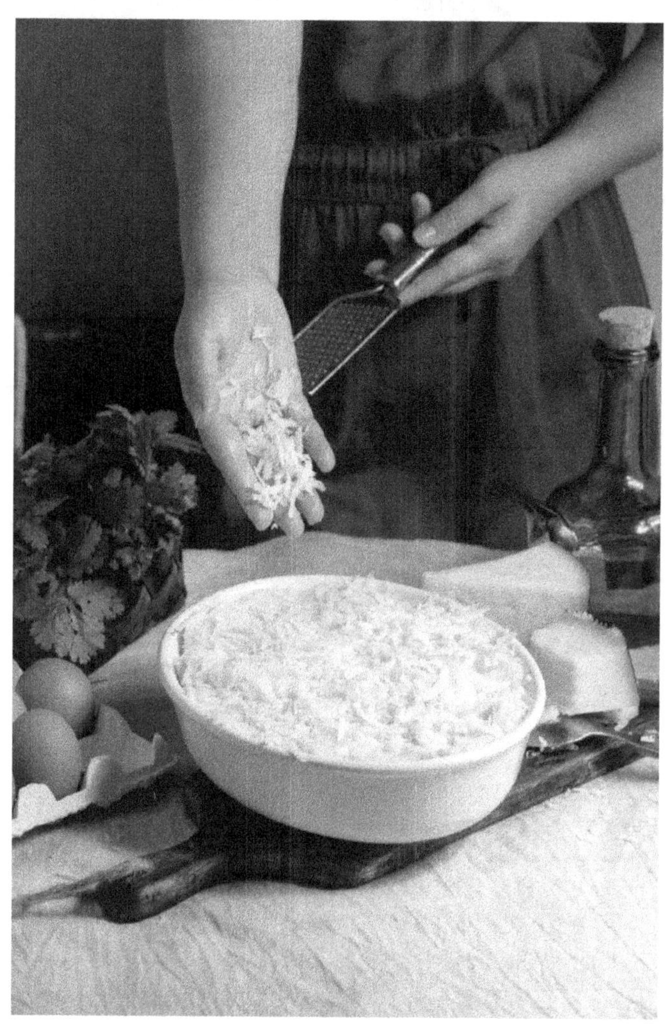

Ingredients:

- 2 large potatoes, peeled and cubed
- 1/4 cup milk
- 2 tbsp butter
- 1/4 cup grated cheese
- Salt to taste

Instructions:

1. Boil the potatoes in water until they are very soft, about 15 minutes.
2. Drain the potatoes and mash them with milk and butter until smooth.
3. Stir in the grated cheese and salt until well combined.
4. Transfer the mixture to a baking dish and spread evenly.
5. Bake in a preheated oven at 350°F (175°C) for 20 minutes, or until heated through and the top is slightly golden.
6. Serve warm, ensuring the bake is soft and easy to spoon for Dysphagia Level 2.

Nutritional Data:
Calories: 350 | Protein: 10g | Carbohydrates: 45g | Fat: 15g | Fiber: 3g | Sugar: 3g

68. Soft Vegetable Risotto

Preparation Time: 10 minutes | Cooking Time: 30 minutes

Ingredients:

- 1/2 cup Arborio rice
- 2 cups vegetable broth
- 1/2 cup zucchini, finely chopped
- 1/2 cup peas
- 1/4 cup grated Parmesan cheese
- Salt to taste

Instructions:

1. In a saucepan, bring 1 cup of vegetable broth to a simmer.
2. Add the Arborio rice and stir continuously until the broth is absorbed.
3. Gradually add the remaining broth, one cup at a time, allowing the rice to absorb the liquid before adding more.
4. When the rice is halfway cooked, add the zucchini and peas.
5. Continue cooking until the rice and vegetables are soft and the risotto has a creamy texture.
6. Stir in the grated Parmesan cheese and season with salt.
7. Before serving, gently mash the risotto to ensure all vegetables are soft enough for Dysphagia Level 2 compliance.

Nutritional Data:
Calories: 380 | Protein: 10g | Carbohydrates: 60g | Fat: 10g | Fiber: 4g | Sugar: 4g

69. Tender Beef Stroganoff

Preparation Time: 15 minutes | Cooking Time: 1 hour

Ingredients:

- 4 oz tender beef cuts, thinly sliced
- 1/2 cup sour cream
- 1/2 cup mushrooms, finely chopped
- 1/4 cup onion, finely chopped
- 1 cup soft noodles or mashed potatoes
- Salt to taste

Instructions:

1. In a skillet, sauté the onion and mushrooms until soft.
2. Add the thinly sliced beef to the skillet and cook until tender.
3. Stir in the sour cream to make a creamy sauce, then reduce the heat and simmer for a few minutes.
4. Prepare the noodles according to package instructions until very

soft, or make mashed potatoes with a very smooth consistency.

5. Serve the beef stroganoff over the soft noodles or mashed potatoes.
6. Ensure the beef is tender and the overall texture is suitable for Dysphagia Level 2 compliance before serving.

Nutritional Data:

Calories: 400 | Protein: 25g | Carbohydrates: 30g | Fat: 20g | Fiber: 2g | Sugar: 3g

70. Soft-Cooked Chicken and Vegetable Pie

Preparation Time: 20 minutes | Cooking Time: 30 minutes

Ingredients:

- 4 oz cooked chicken, finely minced
- 1/2 cup mixed vegetables (carrots, peas), cooked and finely chopped
- 1/2 cup creamy sauce (can use a prepared cream of chicken soup)
- 1 soft pastry crust, pre-cooked (optional)
- 1/2 cup mashed potato, very smooth (if not using pastry)

Instructions:

1. Preheat your oven to 350°F (175°C) if using a pastry crust.
2. In a mixing bowl, combine the finely minced chicken, soft-cooked and finely chopped vegetables, and creamy sauce.
3. If using a soft pastry crust, lay the crust in a small baking dish. Pour the chicken and vegetable mixture into the crust.
4. If not using pastry, place the chicken and vegetable mixture in

the baking dish and top with a layer of very smooth mashed potato.

5. Bake in the preheated oven for 20-25 minutes if using pastry, or just heat through if topped with mashed potato.
6. Ensure the filling is moist and the pastry or potato topping is soft enough to meet Dysphagia Level 2 compliance before serving.

Nutritional Data:

Calories: 350 | Protein: 25g | Carbohydrates: 35g | Fat: 15g | Fiber: 4g | Sugar: 3g

LEVEL3 RECIPES

71. Moist Chicken Parmesan

Preparation Time: 15 minutes | Cooking Time: 30 minutes

Ingredients:

- 4 oz chicken breast, pounded to even thickness
- 1/4 cup soft breadcrumbs
- 1/2 cup marinara sauce
- 1/4 cup shredded mozzarella cheese
- Salt and pepper to taste

Instructions:

1. Preheat the oven to 375°F (190°C).
2. Season the chicken breast with salt and pepper and coat it lightly with soft breadcrumbs.
3. Place the chicken in a baking dish and bake for 20 minutes.
4. Remove the chicken from the oven, and top with marinara sauce and mozzarella cheese.

5. Return to the oven and bake for another 10 minutes until the cheese is melted and bubbly.
6. Let the chicken cool slightly, then cut into small, soft pieces that comply with Dysphagia Level 3 requirements.
7. Serve warm, ensuring the chicken is moist and easy to swallow.

Nutritional Data:
Calories: 300 | Protein: 30g | Carbohydrates: 20g | Fat: 10g | Fiber: 2g | Sugar: 5g

72. Soft Shepherd's Pie

Preparation Time: 20 minutes | Cooking Time: 30 minutes

Ingredients:

- 4 oz ground lamb or beef
- 1/2 cup carrots, finely chopped and cooked until soft
- 1/2 cup peas, cooked until soft
- 1 cup mashed potatoes, made smooth
- Salt and pepper to taste

Instructions:

1. Preheat the oven to 375°F (190°C).
2. Cook the ground meat over medium heat until it's browned and crumbly. Drain any excess fat.
3. Mix the cooked meat with the soft carrots and peas, season with salt and pepper, and place in a baking dish.
4. Top the meat and vegetable mixture with a layer of smooth mashed potatoes.
5. Bake in the preheated oven for 20 minutes until the pie is heated through and the top is slightly golden.
6. Serve warm, ensuring the ground meat is tender and the vegetables are soft to meet Dysphagia Level 3 compliance.

Nutritional Data:
Calories: 400 | Protein: 24g | Carbohydrates: 35g | Fat: 18g | Fiber: 5g | Sugar: 4g

73. Tender Baked Fish Fillet

Preparation Time: 5 minutes | Cooking Time: 15 minutes

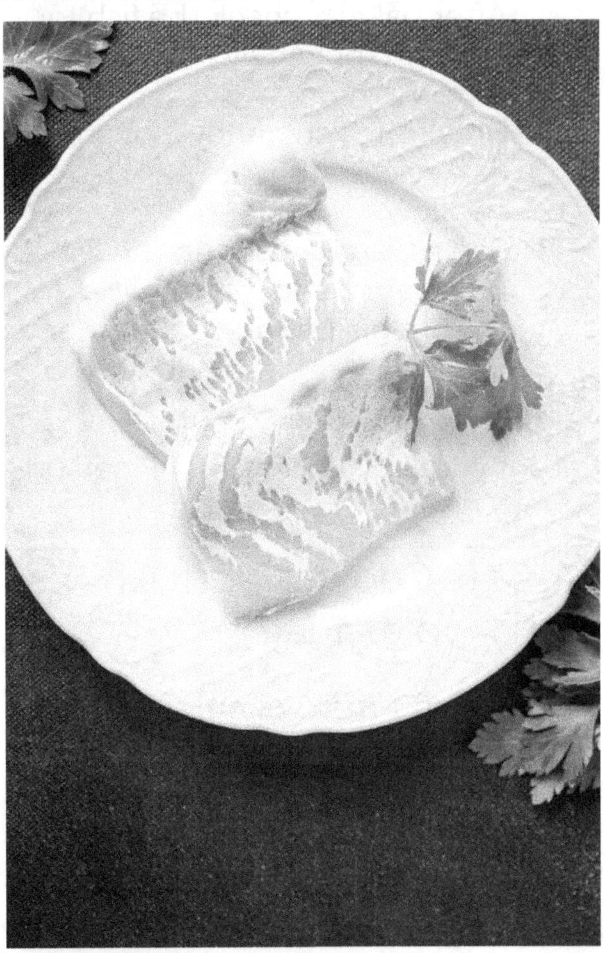

Ingredients:

- 4 oz white fish fillet (cod or tilapia)
- 1 tbsp olive oil
- 1 tsp lemon juice

- 1 tsp chopped fresh herbs (such as dill or parsley)
- Salt and pepper to taste

Instructions:

1. Preheat the oven to 375°F (190°C).
2. Place the fish fillet on a baking sheet lined with parchment paper.
3. Drizzle with olive oil and lemon juice, then season with herbs, salt, and pepper.
4. Bake for 15 minutes or until the fish is cooked through and flakes easily with a fork.
5. After baking, check the fish for any hard or chewy parts and remove them.
6. Break the fish gently into small, flaky pieces that are easy to swallow.
7. Serve warm, ensuring the fish is moist and tender to meet Dysphagia Level 3 requirements.

Nutritional Data:

Calories: 120 | Protein: 23g | Carbohydrates: 0g | Fat: 4g | Fiber: 0g | Sugar: 0g

74. Soft-Cooked Pork Chops with Applesauce

Preparation Time: 5 minutes | Cooking Time: 25 minutes

Ingredients:

- 4 oz pork chops, boneless
- 1/2 cup unsweetened applesauce
- Salt and mild seasoning to taste
- 1 tbsp olive oil

Instructions:

1. Preheat the oven to 350°F (175°C).
2. Season the pork chops with salt and mild seasoning.
3. Heat olive oil in a pan over medium heat and sear the pork chops on both sides until golden.
4. Transfer the pork chops to a baking dish and cover with foil.
5. Bake for 20-25 minutes or until the pork chops are very tender.
6. Let the pork chops rest, then check their tenderness, ensuring no tough or chewy parts remain.
7. Serve the pork chops with a side of smooth applesauce, cutting the meat into small, manageable pieces for easy swallowing.
8. Ensure that the overall texture is appropriate for Dysphagia Level 3 compliance.

Nutritional Data:

Calories: 250 | Protein: 22g | Carbohydrates: 15g | Fat: 10g | Fiber: 1g | Sugar: 12g

75. Creamy Tuna and Noodle Casserole

Preparation Time: 10 minutes | Cooking Time: 25 minutes

Ingredients:

- 4 oz canned tuna, drained
- 1 cup cooked egg noodles
- 1/2 cup cream of mushroom soup
- 1/4 cup peas, cooked until very soft
- Salt and pepper to taste

Instructions:

1. Preheat the oven to 350°F (175°C).
2. In a bowl, flake the tuna with a fork and mix with the cooked egg noodles, cream of mushroom soup, and soft peas.
3. Season with salt and pepper to taste.

4. Transfer the mixture to a baking dish and spread evenly.
5. Bake for 25 minutes or until the casserole is heated through and the top is slightly golden.
6. Before serving, check that the casserole's texture is uniformly soft and moist, breaking down any larger pieces of noodle or tuna to ensure compliance with Dysphagia Level 3 requirements.

Nutritional Data:
Calories: 330 | Protein: 25g | Carbohydrates: 35g | Fat: 9g | Fiber: 3g | Sugar: 2g

76. Soft Roasted Turkey with Gravy

Preparation Time: 20 minutes | Cooking Time: Depends on the size of the turkey

Ingredients:

- 4 oz turkey, cooked until very tender
- 1/2 cup broth (used for roasting)
- Herbs like thyme and sage for seasoning
- 1 tbsp flour or cornstarch (for the gravy)
- Salt and pepper to taste

Instructions:

1. Preheat the oven to the appropriate temperature for the size of the turkey you are cooking.
2. Season the turkey with herbs, salt, and pepper, and roast in the oven using broth to keep it moist, until the turkey reaches an internal temperature of 165°F (74°C).
3. Once the turkey is cooked and very tender, remove it from the oven and let it rest.
4. To make the gravy, pour the juices from the roasting pan into a saucepan, and thicken them with flour or cornstarch to make a smooth gravy.
5. Cut the turkey into very small, soft pieces.
6. Serve the turkey with the gravy, ensuring both the turkey and gravy have a soft, smooth consistency suitable for Dysphagia Level 3.

Nutritional Data:
Calories: 280 | Protein: 25g | Carbohydrates: 10g | Fat: 15g | Fiber: 0.5g | Sugar: 0g

77. Slow-Cooked Beef Goulash

Preparation Time: 20 minutes | Cooking Time: 8 hours (slow cooker on low)

Ingredients:

- 4 oz beef stew meat, cut into small cubes
- 1/2 onion, finely chopped
- 1/2 bell pepper, finely chopped
- 1 cup tomatoes, diced
- 1 tsp paprika
- Salt and pepper to taste
- 1 cup beef broth

Instructions:

1. Place the beef, onion, bell pepper, tomatoes, paprika, salt, pepper, and beef broth into a slow cooker.
2. Set the slow cooker to low and cook for 8 hours, or until the beef is extremely tender.

3. Once cooked, transfer the goulash to a blender and blend until it reaches a smooth consistency.
4. If necessary, add additional beef broth to achieve the desired thickness for Dysphagia Level 3 compliance.
5. Taste and adjust the seasoning as needed.
6. Serve warm, ensuring the goulash is smooth and uniform without any chunks.

Nutritional Data:
Calories: 350 | Protein: 30g | Carbohydrates: 20g | Fat: 15g | Fiber: 3g | Sugar: 5g

LEVEL4 RECIPES

78. Tender Grilled Chicken with Soft Herb Polenta

Preparation Time: 10 minutes | Cooking Time: 30 minutes

Ingredients:

- 4 oz chicken breast
- 1/2 cup polenta (cornmeal)
- 2 cups chicken broth
- 1 tsp fresh herbs (rosemary or thyme), finely chopped
- Salt and pepper to taste

Instructions:

1. Grill or bake the chicken breast until it reaches an internal temperature of 165°F (74°C) and is fully cooked and tender. Let it cool and then cut it into small, tender pieces.
2. In a saucepan, bring the chicken broth to a boil. Gradually whisk in the polenta and the herbs.

3. Reduce the heat to low and continue to cook, stirring regularly, until the polenta is soft and creamy about 20-30 minutes.
4. Season the polenta with salt and pepper.
5. Serve the chicken over the soft polenta, ensuring both are moist and in small enough pieces to comply with Dysphagia Level 4 requirements.

Nutritional Data:
Calories: 350 | Protein: 30g | Carbohydrates: 40g | Fat: 5g | Fiber: 2g | Sugar: 1g

79. Moist Meatballs in Marinara Sauce

Preparation Time: 15 minutes | Cooking Time: 20 minutes

Ingredients:

- 4 oz ground beef or turkey
- 1/4 cup breadcrumbs
- 1 egg, beaten
- 1 cup marinara sauce
- Salt and pepper to taste

Instructions:

1. Preheat the oven to 375°F (190°C).
2. In a bowl, mix the ground meat, breadcrumbs, egg, salt, and pepper.
3. Form the mixture into small meatballs.
4. Place the meatballs on a baking sheet and bake for 15-20 minutes until they are cooked through and tender.
5. Warm the marinara sauce in a saucepan.

6. Add the cooked meatballs to the marinara sauce and let them simmer for a few minutes.
7. Before serving, ensure the meatballs and sauce have a soft, smooth consistency appropriate for Dysphagia Level 4 compliance.

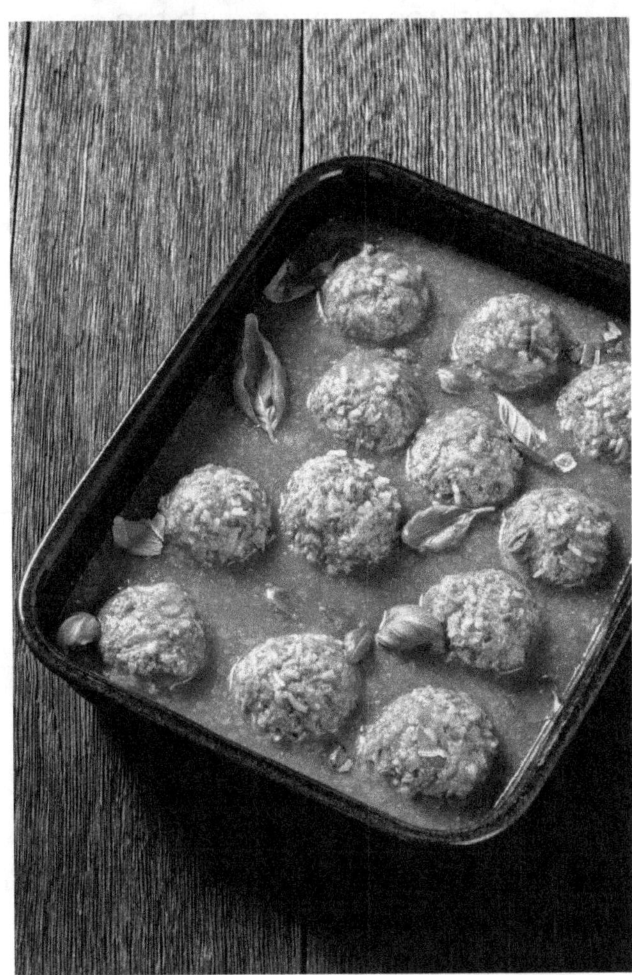

Nutritional Data:
Calories: 400 | Protein: 25g | Carbohydrates: 25g | Fat: 20g | Fiber: 3g | Sugar: 8g

80. Flaky Baked Salmon with Dill Sauce

Preparation Time: 5 minutes | Cooking Time: 15 minutes

Ingredients:

- 4 oz salmon fillet
- 1 tbsp fresh dill, finely chopped
- 1 tsp lemon juice
- 1/4 cup cream or plain yogurt
- Salt and pepper to taste

Instructions:

1. Preheat the oven to 400°F (200°C).
2. Season the salmon with salt and pepper, and place it on a baking sheet lined with parchment paper.
3. Bake for about 12-15 minutes, or until the salmon is cooked through and flakes easily with a fork.
4. While the salmon is baking, mix the dill, lemon juice, and cream or yogurt to create the dill sauce.
5. Once the salmon is done, let it cool slightly and check for any bones. Flake the salmon gently.
6. Serve the salmon topped with the smooth dill sauce, ensuring the salmon is moist and flaky to comply with Dysphagia Level 4 requirements.

Nutritional Data:
Calories: 300 | Protein: 23g | Carbohydrates: 2g | Fat: 22g | Fiber: 0g | Sugar: 1g

81. Slow-Cooked Pulled Pork with Soft Rolls

Preparation Time: 20 minutes | Cooking Time: 8 hours (slow cooker on low)

Ingredients:

- 4 oz pork shoulder
- 1/4 cup barbecue sauce
- Spices (such as smoked paprika, and garlic powder) to taste

- 1 soft dinner roll

Instructions:

1. Season the pork shoulder with spices.
2. Place the pork in a slow cooker and cook on low for 8 hours or until very tender.
3. Once the pork is cooked, shred it with two forks, ensuring there are no tough pieces.
4. Mix the shredded pork with barbecue sauce, heating through if necessary.
5. Serve the pulled pork alongside or on top of a soft dinner roll, ensuring both the pork and roll are moist and soft for Dysphagia Level 4 compliance.

Nutritional Data:
Calories: 500 | Protein: 30g | Carbohydrates: 40g | Fat: 25g | Fiber: 1g | Sugar: 20g

82. Soft-Cooked Beef Stroganoff over Egg Noodles

Preparation Time: 10 minutes | Cooking Time: 20 minutes

Ingredients:

- 4 oz thinly sliced beef
- 1/2 cup mushrooms, finely chopped
- 1/2 cup sour cream
- 1 cup cooked egg noodles
- Salt and pepper to taste

Instructions:

1. Sauté the beef in a pan over medium heat until it is just cooked through and tender.
2. Add the mushrooms to the pan and cook until they are soft.

3. Reduce the heat and stir in the sour cream to make a creamy sauce. Heat gently, being careful not to boil.
4. Cook the egg noodles according to the package instructions until they are very soft, then drain.
5. Combine the beef and mushroom sauce with the egg noodles, ensuring the beef is cut into small, manageable pieces.
6. Season with salt and pepper to taste and serve warm.
7. Check the final dish to ensure it meets the softness required for Dysphagia Level 4 compliance.

Nutritional Data:
Calories: 400 | Protein: 30g | Carbohydrates: 30g | Fat: 18g | Fiber: 2g | Sugar: 3g

83. Baked Lasagna with Soft Cheese Filling

Preparation Time: 15 minutes | Cooking Time: 45 minutes

Ingredients:

- 2 cooked lasagna noodles, cut to fit the dish
- 1/2 cup ricotta or cottage cheese
- 1/4 cup shredded mozzarella cheese
- 1 cup marinara sauce
- Salt and pepper to taste

Instructions:

1. Preheat the oven to 375°F (190°C).
2. Spread a thin layer of marinara sauce on the bottom of a small baking dish.
3. Place one layer of the soft-cooked lasagna noodles over the sauce.

4. Spread the ricotta or cottage cheese over the noodles, then add another layer of marinara sauce.
5. Repeat the layers, finishing with a layer of marinara sauce and topping with shredded mozzarella cheese.
6. Cover with foil and bake for about 30 minutes. Remove the foil and bake for an additional 15 minutes until the cheese is melted and the dish is heated through.
7. Let the lasagna cool slightly, then check the tenderness of the pasta and cheese to ensure they are soft enough for Dysphagia Level 4 compliance.
8. Serve warm, cutting into small, manageable portions.

Nutritional Data:

Calories: 450 | Protein: 25g | Carbohydrates: 35g | Fat: 22g | Fiber: 3g | Sugar: 6g

84. Creamy Vegetable Curry with Soft Rice

Preparation Time: 15 minutes | Cooking Time: 30 minutes

Ingredients:

- 1/2 cup assorted vegetables (like carrots, peas, and potatoes), finely chopped
- 1 tsp curry powder (mild)
- 1/2 cup coconut milk
- 1 cup rice, cooked until very soft
- Salt to taste

Instructions:

1. Cook the rice with extra water to ensure it's softer than usual, then set aside.
2. In a pan, add a little water and the finely chopped vegetables. Cook over medium heat until the vegetables are very soft.
3. Stir in the curry powder and cook for another minute to release the flavors.
4. Pour in the coconut milk and bring the mixture to a gentle simmer. Cook until everything is well combined and the vegetables are soft enough to meet Dysphagia Level 4 requirements.
5. Season with salt to taste.
6. Serve the vegetable curry over the soft-cooked rice, ensuring both the curry and rice are soft and tender.

Nutritional Data:

Calories: 350 | Protein: 6g | Carbohydrates: 60g | Fat: 10g | Fiber: 5g | Sugar: 3g

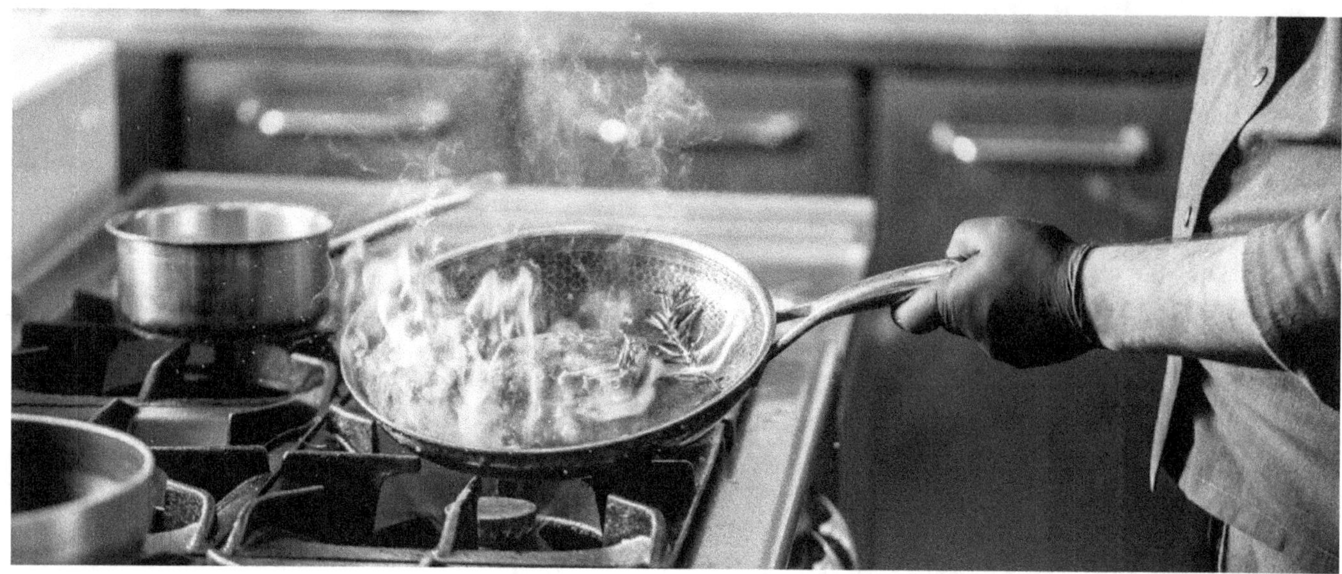

Sides and Snacks

Recognizing the importance of diversity in a dysphagia diet, we've compiled a range of recipes that add excitement and nutritional value to your daily eating routine, all the while being mindful of swallowing safety.

Sides and snacks are essential in any diet, offering an opportunity to increase calorie and nutrient intake, especially important in a dysphagia diet. Here, we present a collection of recipes that range from smooth and creamy to soft and easily chewable, ensuring there's something suitable for every level of dysphagia.

For those following a Pureed Diet (Level 1), we have a selection of smooth, velvety side dishes and snacks. Think whipped potatoes, pureed fruit compotes, and smooth vegetable dips, all designed to be both easy to swallow and full of flavor.

Moving to the Soft and Well-Cooked level (Level 2), the texture becomes slightly more varied. Recipes like soft-cooked vegetable salads, moist rice dishes, and tender, flaky pastries offer a gentle transition from pureed to more solid foods.

As we progress to Advanced Textures (Level 3), sides and snacks include softly cooked, diced vegetables, moist grain salads, and soft, ripe fruit pieces, providing a greater variety of textures and flavors while still focusing on ease of swallowing.

For individuals on the Regular Diet with Modifications (Level 4), the recipes expand further to include a wider array of side dishes and snacks, like soft-roasted vegetables, gentle stir-fries, and easy-to-chew fruit bars, ensuring they are prepared in a way that is mindful of dysphagia requirements.

Each recipe in this chapter not only complements your main meals but also serves as a standalone snack, perfect for satisfying hunger between meals. We understand the significance of sides and snacks in keeping the diet both interesting and nutritionally balanced.

LEVEL 1 RECIPES

85. Smooth Mashed Butternut Squash

Preparation Time: 10 minutes | Cooking Time: 20 minutes

Ingredients:

- 1 cup butternut squash, peeled and cubed
- A pinch of cinnamon
- 1 tbsp butter or cream
- Salt to taste

Instructions:

1. Steam the butternut squash cubes until they are very soft, about 20 minutes.
2. Transfer the soft squash to a blending bowl, add cinnamon, butter or cream, and salt.
3. Use an immersion blender or regular blender to puree the mixture until it's completely smooth, with no lumps.
4. Check the consistency and add a little water or additional cream if needed to reach a velvety texture.
5. Serve warm, ensuring the puree is uniform and meets Dysphagia Level 1 compliance.

Nutritional Data:

Calories: 120 | Protein: 1g | Carbohydrates: 15g | Fat: 7g | Fiber: 2g | Sugar: 3g

86. Creamy Pureed Peas

Preparation Time: 5 minutes | Cooking Time: 10 minutes

Ingredients:

- 1 cup green peas, fresh or frozen
- 2 tbsp cream
- Salt and pepper to taste

Instructions:

1. If using fresh peas, steam them until they are very soft, about 10 minutes. If using frozen, cook according to package instructions until soft.
2. Place the soft peas in a blending bowl, and add cream, salt, and pepper.
3. Blend the peas with an immersion blender or in a regular blender until completely smooth.
4. Adjust the seasoning to taste and check the consistency, adding more cream if necessary for a smooth, creamy texture.
5. Serve warm, ensuring the pureed peas are smooth and suitable for Dysphagia Level 1 compliance.

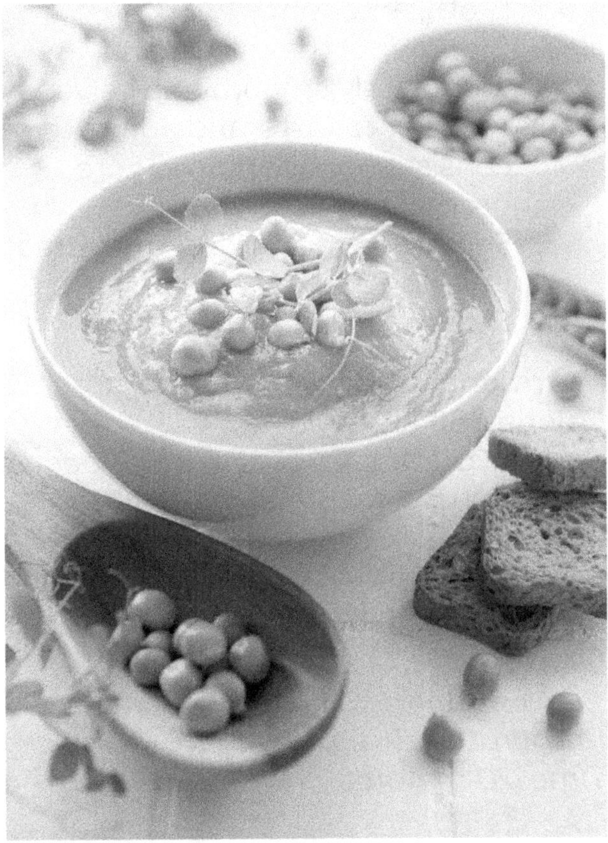

Nutritional Data:
Calories: 150 | Protein: 5g |
Carbohydrates: 13g | Fat: 9g | Fiber: 4g |
Sugar: 4g

87. Velvety Carrot and Ginger Puree

Preparation Time: 10 minutes | Cooking Time: 20 minutes

Ingredients:

- 1 cup carrots, peeled and chopped
- 1/2 tsp fresh ginger, grated
- 1 cup vegetable broth
- 1 tsp honey
- Salt to taste

Instructions:

1. Steam the carrots until they are very soft, about 20 minutes.
2. In a blender, combine the soft carrots, grated ginger, vegetable broth, and honey.
3. Blend until the mixture is completely smooth and velvety.
4. Add salt to taste, and adjust the consistency by adding more broth if needed.
5. Serve warm, ensuring the puree is uniform and complies with Dysphagia Level 1 standards.

Nutritional Data:
Calories: 80 | Protein: 1g |
Carbohydrates: 18g | Fat: 0.2g | Fiber: 4g | Sugar: 10g

88. Silken Pear and Apple Compote

Preparation Time: 10 minutes | Cooking Time: 20 minutes

Ingredients:

- 1 medium pear, peeled and chopped
- 1 medium apple, peeled and chopped
- 1/2 tsp cinnamon
- 1/4 cup apple juice

Instructions:

1. In a saucepan, add the chopped pear and apple with the apple juice and cinnamon.
2. Cook over medium heat until the fruits are very soft, about 20 minutes.
3. Transfer the soft fruits to a blender and puree until smooth.
4. If necessary, add a little more apple juice to achieve the desired consistency.
5. Serve warm or chilled, ensuring the compote is smooth and adheres to Dysphagia Level 1 requirements.

Nutritional Data:
Calories: 150 | Protein: 0.5g |
Carbohydrates: 38g | Fat: 0.3g | Fiber: 5g | Sugar: 28g

89. Smooth Avocado Puree

Preparation Time: 5 minutes | Cooking Time: 0 minutes

Ingredients:

- 1 ripe avocado
- 1 tsp lemon juice
- Salt to taste

Instructions:

1. Cut the avocado in half, remove the pit, and scoop out the flesh.

2. Place the avocado in a blender, and add lemon juice, and a pinch of salt.
3. Blend until the mixture is completely smooth, with no lumps or chunks.
4. Taste and adjust the seasoning if necessary.
5. Serve immediately or store in an airtight container with plastic wrap pressed onto the surface to prevent browning.
6. Ensure the puree maintains a smooth consistency that meets Dysphagia Level 1 standards.

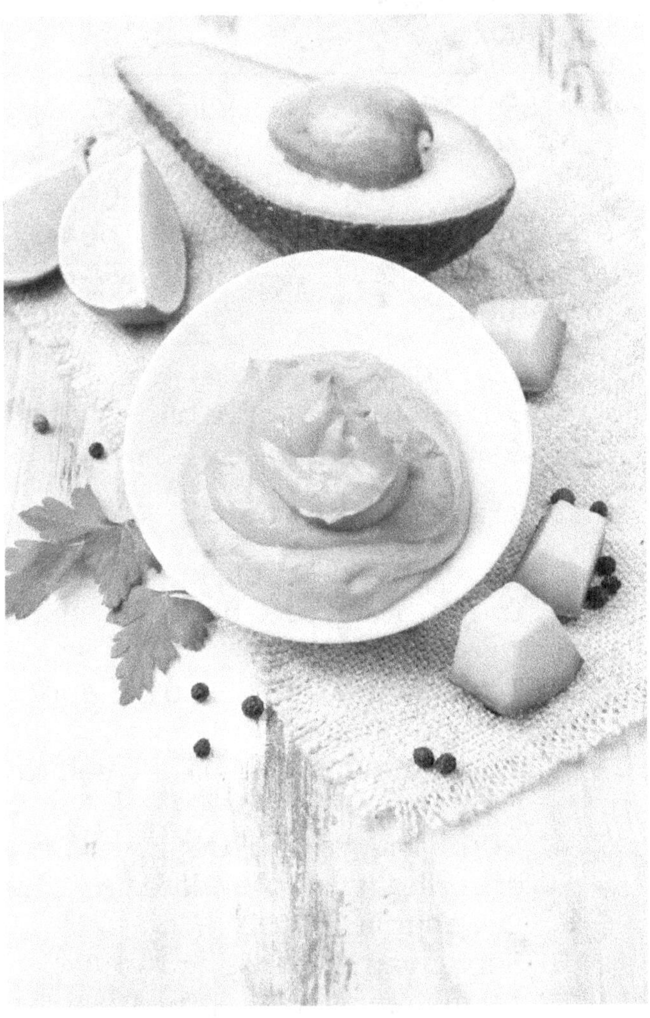

Nutritional Data:
Calories: 230 | Protein: 3g | Carbohydrates: 12g | Fat: 21g | Fiber: 9g | Sugar: 1g

90. Silken Tofu and Berry Compote

Preparation Time: 5 minutes | Cooking Time: 10 minutes

Ingredients:

- 1/2 cup silken tofu
- 1/2 cup mixed berries (like strawberries and blueberries, fresh or frozen)
- 1 tablespoon sugar or honey (optional, adjust to taste)
- 1/4 cup water

Instructions:

1. In a small saucepan, combine berries, sugar/honey (if using), and water. Simmer over low heat until the berries are soft and the mixture has a sauce-like consistency, about 8-10 minutes.
2. Allow the berry mixture to cool slightly, then blend until smooth. Strain if necessary to ensure no seeds or skins are left.
3. Place silken tofu in a bowl. If desired, blend the tofu to ensure it's completely smooth.
4. Pour the berry compote over the silken tofu. Serve immediately.

Nutritional Data:
Calories: 150 | Protein: 5 g | Fat: 3.5 g | Carbohydrates: 25.6 g | Fiber: 2.5 g

91. Creamy Mashed Cauliflower

Preparation Time: 10 minutes | Cooking Time: 10 minutes

Ingredients:

- 1 cup cauliflower florets
- 1 garlic clove, minced

- 2 tbsp cream
- Salt and pepper to taste

Instructions:

1. Steam the cauliflower florets until they are very soft, about 10 minutes.
2. In a blender or food processor, combine the steamed cauliflower, minced garlic, cream, salt, and pepper.
3. Blend until the mixture is completely smooth and creamy, with no lumps.
4. Taste and adjust the seasoning if necessary.
5. Serve warm, ensuring the mashed cauliflower maintains a smooth consistency suitable for Dysphagia Level 1.

Nutritional Data:
Calories: 100 | Protein: 2g | Carbohydrates: 8g | Fat: 7g | Fiber: 3g | Sugar: 3g

LEVEL2 RECIPES

92. Soft-Cooked Mashed Potatoes

Preparation Time: 10 minutes | Cooking Time: 20 minutes

Ingredients:

- 2 large potatoes, peeled and cubed
- 2 tbsp butter
- 1/4 cup cream
- Salt to taste

Instructions:

1. Boil the potato cubes in water until they are very soft, about 20 minutes.
2. Drain the potatoes and return them to the pot.
3. Add butter, cream, and salt to the potatoes.
4. Mash the potatoes until they are smooth but still have a slightly textured consistency appropriate for Dysphagia Level 2.
5. Serve warm, ensuring the mashed potatoes are soft and not too thick or sticky.

Nutritional Data:
Calories: 300 | Protein: 4g | Carbohydrates: 35g | Fat: 17g | Fiber: 3g | Sugar: 2g

93. Tender Steamed Broccoli Puree

Preparation Time: 5 minutes | Cooking Time: 10 minutes
Ingredients:

- 1 cup broccoli florets
- 1 tbsp butter or olive oil
- Salt to taste

Instructions:

1. Steam the broccoli florets until they are very soft, about 10 minutes.
2. Transfer the broccoli to a blender or food processor.
3. Add butter or olive oil and salt to the broccoli.
4. Puree the mixture until smooth, ensuring it's appropriate for Dysphagia Level 2.
5. Serve warm, adjusting the consistency with a little water if necessary to ensure it's not too thick.

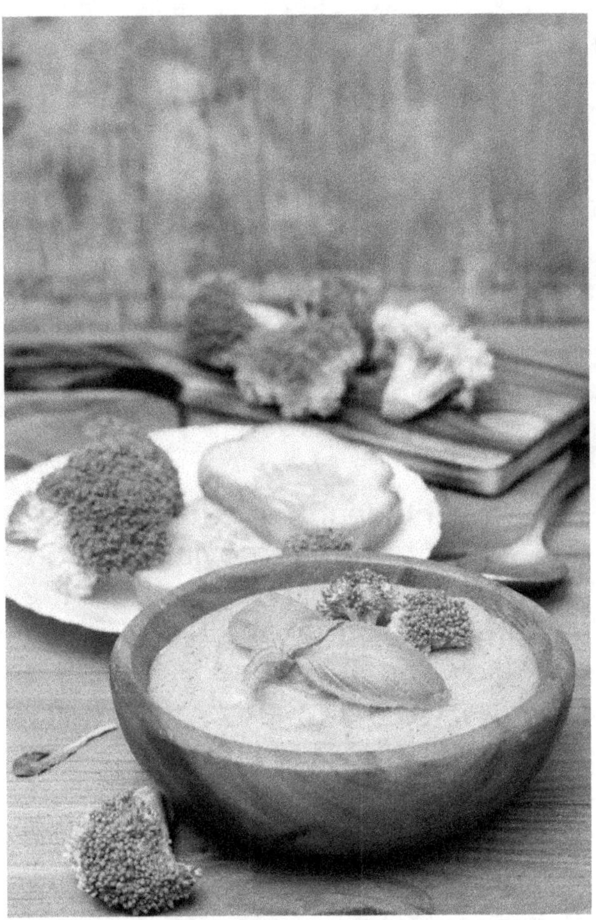

Nutritional Data:
Calories: 100 | Protein: 3g |
Carbohydrates: 8g | Fat: 7g | Fiber: 3g |
Sugar: 2g

94. Honeyed Pear Puree

Preparation Time: 5 minutes | Cooking Time: 30 minutes

Ingredients:

- 1 ripe pear, peeled, cored, and chopped
- 2 tablespoons water
- 1 tablespoon honey (or to taste)
- A pinch of ground cinnamon (optional)

Instructions:

1. In a small saucepan, combine the chopped pear and water. Cook over medium heat until the pear is very soft, about 8-10 minutes.
2. Remove from heat and let it cool slightly. Blend the pear using a hand blender or food processor until it reaches a smooth, consistent puree.
3. Stir in the honey and a pinch of cinnamon (if using), mixing well to ensure a smooth texture.
4. If the puree is too thick, you can add a little more water to reach the desired consistency.
5. The puree can be served warm or refrigerated and served chilled, depending on preference.

Nutritional Data:
Calories: 220 (without cheese) | Protein: 4g | Carbohydrates: 40g | Fat: 2g (without cheese) | Fiber: 4g | Sugar: 6g (if using milk)

95. Soft Baked Apple Slices

Preparation Time: 10 minutes | Cooking Time: 25 minutes

Ingredients:

- 1 large apple, cored and sliced
- 1/2 tsp cinnamon
- 1 tbsp sugar or honey

Instructions:

1. Preheat the oven to 350°F (175°C).
2. Arrange the apple slices in a single layer on a baking sheet.
3. Sprinkle with cinnamon and drizzle with sugar or honey.
4. Bake in the preheated oven for 25 minutes or until the apples are soft and tender.
5. Once baked, check to ensure the apple slices are soft enough to mash with minimal effort.
6. Serve warm, ensuring the apples are easy to chew for Dysphagia Level 2 compliance.

Nutritional Data:
Calories: 90 | Protein: 0g |
Carbohydrates: 24g | Fat: 0g | Fiber: 4g |
Sugar: 19g

96. Moist Pumpkin Custard

Preparation Time: 10 minutes | Cooking Time: 30 minutes

Ingredients:

- 1/2 cup pumpkin puree
- 1 egg
- 1/2 cup milk
- 2 tbsp sugar
- 1/2 tsp pumpkin pie spice

Instructions:

1. Preheat the oven to 350°F (175°C).
2. In a bowl, whisk together the pumpkin puree, egg, milk, sugar, and pumpkin pie spice until smooth.
3. Pour the mixture into a small baking dish or ramekin.
4. Place the baking dish in a larger pan and fill the pan with hot water to about halfway up the sides of the dish (water bath).
5. Bake for 30 minutes or until the custard is set.
6. Remove from the oven and allow to cool slightly. Check to ensure the custard is moist and spoonable, with a uniform consistency appropriate for Dysphagia Level 2.

Nutritional Data:
Calories: 180 | Protein: 6g |
Carbohydrates: 25g | Fat: 6g | Fiber: 2g |
Sugar: 22g

97. Soft Pear and Cottage Cheese

Preparation Time: 5 minutes | Cooking Time: 10 minutes

Ingredients:

- 1 ripe pear
- 1/2 cup cottage cheese

Instructions:

1. Peel the pear and cut it into small chunks, removing the core.
2. Steam the pear chunks until they are very soft, about 10 minutes.
3. Allow the pear to cool slightly, then mash it gently with a fork.
4. Serve the soft pear with a side of creamy cottage cheese, ensuring both are at a suitable texture for Dysphagia Level 2.

Nutritional Data:
Calories: 150 | Protein: 14g |
Carbohydrates: 20g | Fat: 2g | Fiber: 3g |
Sugar: 16g

98. Soft Rice Pudding

Preparation Time: 5 minutes | Cooking Time: 25 minutes

Ingredients:

- 1/4 cup uncooked rice
- 1 cup milk
- 2 tbsp sugar
- 1/2 tsp vanilla extract
- A sprinkle of cinnamon

Instructions:

1. In a saucepan, combine rice, milk, and sugar. Cook over medium heat until the mixture comes to a boil.

2. Reduce heat to low, cover, and simmer, stirring occasionally, until the rice is tender and the mixture is creamy, about 20-25 minutes.
3. Remove from heat and stir in vanilla extract.
4. Allow the rice pudding to cool slightly, it should be warm but not hot.
5. Sprinkle with a bit of cinnamon before serving.
6. Ensure the pudding is soft and creamy without any hard rice grains, suitable for Dysphagia Level 2 compliance.

Nutritional Data:
Calories: 200 | Protein: 4g | Carbohydrates: 37g | Fat: 3g | Fiber: 0.5g | Sugar: 18g

LEVEL3 RECIPES

99. Soft-Cooked Carrot and Swede Mash

Preparation Time: 10 minutes | Cooking Time: 20 minutes

Ingredients:

- 1/2 cup carrots, peeled and chopped
- 1/2 cup swede (rutabaga), peeled and chopped
- 1 tbsp butter
- Salt and pepper to taste

Instructions:

1. Boil the carrots and swede in water until they are very soft, about 20 minutes.
2. Drain the vegetables and return them to the pot.
3. Add butter, salt, and pepper.

4. Mash the vegetables until they are soft and well combined with a smooth consistency.
5. Serve warm, checking the texture to ensure it is soft and moist, adhering to Dysphagia Level 3 requirements.

Nutritional Data:
Calories: 120 | Protein: 1g | Carbohydrates: 18g | Fat: 5g | Fiber: 4g | Sugar: 9g

100. Tender Peas and Carrots in Butter

Preparation Time: 5 minutes | Cooking Time: 10 minutes

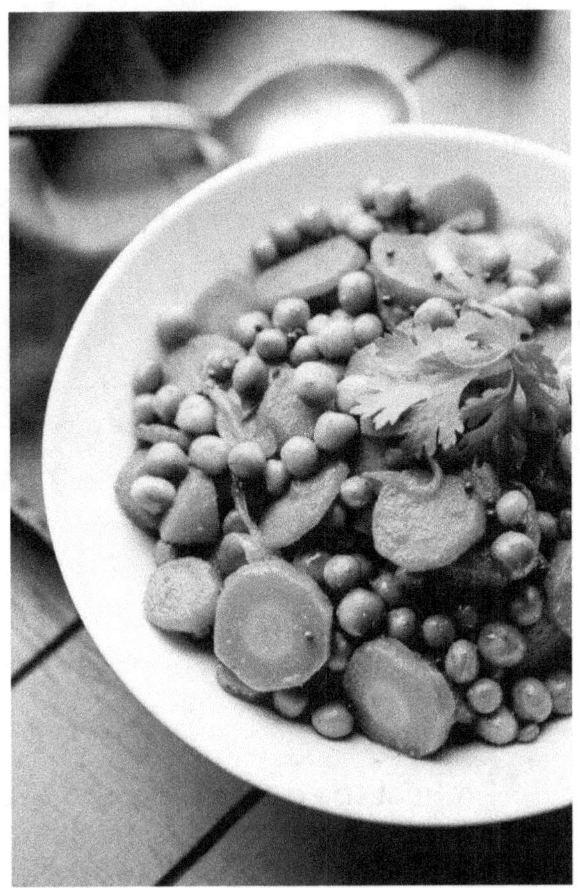

Ingredients:

- 1/2 cup peas, fresh or frozen
- 1/2 cup carrots, diced
- 1 tbsp butter
- Salt to taste

Instructions:

1. Steam the peas and diced carrots until they are very soft about 10 minutes.
2. Once steamed, transfer to a bowl and add butter while they are still hot.
3. Mash the vegetables slightly or leave them whole if they are soft enough to meet Dysphagia Level 3 requirements.
4. Season with salt and mix well to evenly distribute the butter.
5. Serve warm, ensuring the vegetables are tender and coated with butter for ease of swallowing.

Nutritional Data:
Calories: 90 | Protein: 2g | Carbohydrates: 10g | Fat: 5g | Fiber: 3g | Sugar: 4g

101. Moist Zucchini Bread

Preparation Time: 15 minutes | Cooking Time: 45 minutes

Ingredients:

- 1/2 cup grated zucchini
- 1 cup flour
- 1 egg
- 1/2 cup sugar
- 1/2 tsp cinnamon
- 1/4 cup vegetable oil

Instructions:

1. Preheat the oven to 350°F (175°C).
2. In a bowl, mix the flour, sugar, and cinnamon.
3. In another bowl, beat the egg and mix with the vegetable oil and grated zucchini.
4. Combine the wet and dry ingredients and mix until just incorporated.
5. Pour the batter into a greased loaf pan.
6. Bake for 45 minutes or until a toothpick inserted into the center comes out clean.
7. Allow the bread to cool, then cut it into small, moist pieces that comply with Dysphagia Level 3 requirements.
8. Serve slightly warm or at room temperature, ensuring the texture is moist and easy to chew.

Nutritional Data:
Calories: 250 | Protein: 4g | Carbohydrates: 40g | Fat: 9g | Fiber: 1g | Sugar: 20g

102. Creamy Baked Custard

Preparation Time: 10 minutes | Cooking Time: 45 minutes

Ingredients:

- 2 cups milk
- 2 eggs
- 1/4 cup sugar
- 1/2 tsp vanilla extract

Instructions:

1. Preheat the oven to 325°F (165°C).
2. Warm the milk in a saucepan until hot but not boiling.
3. In a bowl, whisk the eggs, sugar, and vanilla extract together.
4. Gradually add the hot milk to the egg mixture, whisking constantly.
5. Pour the mixture into ramekins or a baking dish.
6. Place the ramekins or dish in a large roasting pan and fill the pan with hot water to about halfway up the sides of the ramekins or dish (water bath).

7. Bake for 45 minutes or until the custard is set but still slightly wobbly in the center.
8. Remove from the oven and allow to cool slightly. Ensure the custard is smooth and at the right consistency for Dysphagia Level 3 compliance before serving.

Nutritional Data:
Calories: 180 | Protein: 8g | Carbohydrates: 24g | Fat: 6g | Fiber: 0g | Sugar: 24g

103. Soft Banana Pudding

Preparation Time: 10 minutes | Cooking Time: 5 minutes (plus chilling time)

Ingredients:

- 1 ripe banana, well-mashed
- 1 cup milk
- 2 tbsp sugar
- 1 package vanilla pudding mix (appropriate for 1 cup of milk)

Instructions:

1. In a medium bowl, prepare the vanilla pudding according to the package instructions using 1 cup of milk.
2. Add the sugar to the pudding mixture and stir well.
3. Fold the well-mashed banana into the pudding until well combined.
4. Pour the mixture into a serving dish or individual cups.
5. Refrigerate until the pudding is set, usually about 1 hour.
6. Before serving, check the consistency to ensure that the pudding and banana are soft enough to meet Dysphagia Level 3 standards.

Nutritional Data:
Calories: 200 | Protein: 5g | Carbohydrates: 38g | Fat: 3g | Fiber: 1g | Sugar: 28g

104. Tender Baked Pear Halves

Preparation Time: 5 minutes | Cooking Time: 30 minutes

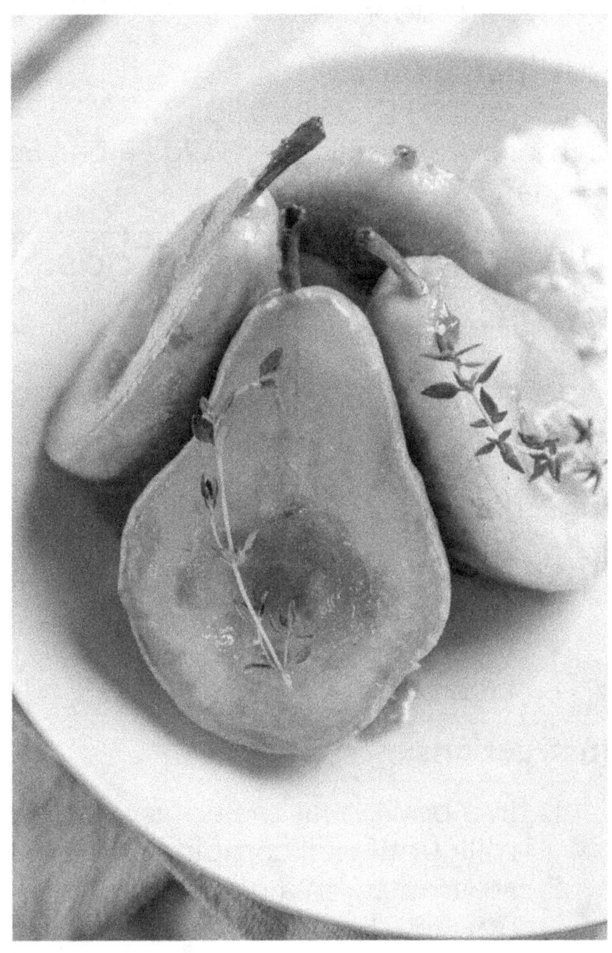

Ingredients:

- 1 large pear, halved and cored
- 1 tbsp honey or maple syrup
- A sprinkle of cinnamon

Instructions:

1. Preheat the oven to 350°F (175°C).
2. Place the pear halves cut side up on a baking dish.

3. Drizzle with honey or maple syrup and sprinkle with cinnamon.
4. Bake in the preheated oven for 30 minutes or until the pears are soft and tender.
5. Once done, allow the pears to cool slightly to ensure they are safe to eat and comply with Dysphagia Level 3 requirements for tenderness.

Nutritional Data:
Calories: 120 | Protein: 0.5g | Carbohydrates: 31g | Fat: 0.2g | Fiber: 5g | Sugar: 25g

105. Fluffy Scrambled Eggs with Cheese

Preparation Time: 2 minutes | Cooking Time: 5 minutes

Ingredients:

- 2 eggs
- 2 tbsp milk
- 1/4 cup shredded cheese
- 1 tsp butter

Instructions:

1. In a bowl, beat the eggs with the milk until well combined.
2. Melt butter in a non-stick pan over low heat.
3. Add the egg mixture to the pan and let it sit undisturbed until it begins to set around the edges.
4. Using a spatula, gently stir the eggs, pushing from the edges to the center.
5. Sprinkle the shredded cheese over the eggs and continue to cook until the eggs are fluffy, moist, and just set.
6. Serve warm, ensuring the eggs are soft and moist, suitable for Dysphagia Level 3 compliance.

Nutritional Data:
Calories: 210 | Protein: 14g | Carbohydrates: 2g | Fat: 16g | Fiber: 0g | Sugar: 2g

LEVEL4 RECIPES

106. Soft Baked Apple and Cinnamon Wedges

Preparation Time: 5 minutes | Cooking Time: 25 minutes

Ingredients:

- 1 large apple, cored and cut into wedges
- 1/2 tsp cinnamon
- 1 tbsp sugar

Instructions:

1. Preheat the oven to 350°F (175°C).
2. Arrange the apple wedges in a single layer on a baking sheet.
3. Sprinkle with cinnamon and sugar.
4. Bake for 25 minutes or until the apples are tender.
5. After baking, test to ensure the apple wedges are soft enough to meet Dysphagia Level 4 requirements.
6. Serve warm, ensuring the apple wedges are easy to chew and swallow.

Nutritional Data:
Calories: 90 | Protein: 0.5g | Carbohydrates: 24g | Fat: 0.2g | Fiber: 4g | Sugar: 19g

107. Creamy Mashed Sweet Potatoes

Preparation Time: 10 minutes | Cooking Time: 20 minutes

Ingredients:

- 1 large sweet potato, peeled and cubed
- 2 tbsp cream
- 1 tbsp butter
- Salt and pepper to taste

Instructions:

1. Boil the sweet potato cubes in water until they are very tender, about 20 minutes.
2. Drain the sweet potatoes and return them to the pot.
3. Add cream, butter, salt, and pepper to the pot.
4. Mash the sweet potatoes until smooth.
5. Serve warm, ensuring the mashed sweet potatoes are soft and well-mashed to comply with Dysphagia Level 4 standards.

Nutritional Data:
Calories: 200 | Protein: 2g | Carbohydrates: 27g | Fat: 9g | Fiber: 4g | Sugar: 6g

108. Tender Steamed Green Beans with Almonds

Preparation Time: 5 minutes | Cooking Time: 10 minutes

Ingredients:

- 1 cup green beans, trimmed
- 1/4 cup almonds, finely chopped and toasted
- 1 tbsp butter
- Salt and pepper to taste

Instructions:

1. Steam the green beans until they are very soft, about 10 minutes.
2. While the green beans are steaming, toast the finely chopped almonds in a dry pan until golden brown, then let them cool.
3. Once the green beans are done, toss them with butter, and season with salt and pepper.
4. Sprinkle the toasted almonds on top just before serving.
5. Ensure the green beans and almonds are soft enough to comply with Dysphagia Level 4 standards. If necessary, chop the green beans into smaller pieces for easy swallowing.

Nutritional Data:
Calories: 150 | Protein: 4g | Carbohydrates: 8g | Fat: 12g | Fiber: 4g | Sugar: 2g

109. Moist Banana Mini-Muffins

Preparation Time: 10 minutes | Cooking Time: 12-15 minutes

Ingredients:

- 1 ripe banana, mashed
- 1 cup flour
- 1/2 cup sugar
- 1 egg
- 1 tsp baking powder

Instructions:

1. Preheat the oven to 350°F (175°C). Grease a mini muffin pan or use paper liners.
2. In a bowl, combine the flour, sugar, and baking powder.

3. In another bowl, mix the mashed banana and egg.
4. Combine the wet and dry ingredients until just mixed.
5. Spoon the batter into the mini muffin pan.
6. Bake for 12-15 minutes or until a toothpick inserted into the center comes out clean.
7. Let the muffins cool, then check for moisture and softness. The muffins should be easy to chew and swallow for Dysphagia Level 4 compliance.

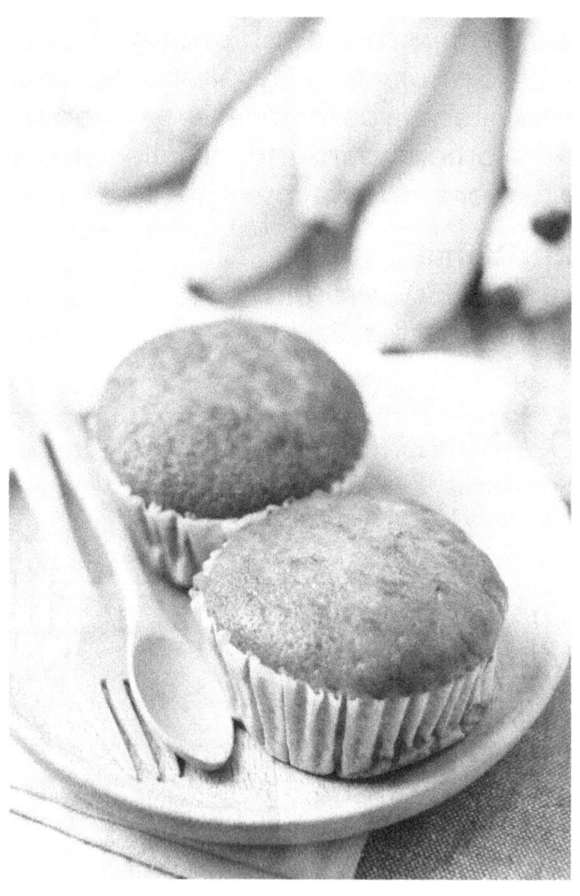

Nutritional Data:
Calories: 100 per mini-muffin | Protein: 2g | Carbohydrates: 18g | Fat: 2g | Fiber: 1g | Sugar: 10g

110. Soft-Cooked Pear Compote

Preparation Time: 5 minutes | Cooking Time: 15 minutes

Ingredients:

- 2 ripe pears, peeled and diced
- 1/4 tsp vanilla extract
- 1 tbsp sugar

Instructions:

1. In a saucepan over medium heat, combine the diced pears, vanilla extract, and sugar.
2. Cook until the pears are very soft and the mixture has thickened into a compote, about 15 minutes.
3. Mash the pears gently with a fork or potato masher to ensure there are no large chunks.
4. Serve warm, ensuring the compote is soft enough to meet Dysphagia Level 4 requirements.

Nutritional Data:
Calories: 100 | Protein: 0.5g | Carbohydrates: 26g | Fat: 0.2g | Fiber: 4g | Sugar: 20g

111. Creamy Rice and Cheese Bake

Preparation Time: 10 minutes | Cooking Time: 20 minutes

Ingredients:

- 1 cup cooked rice
- 1 tbsp flour
- 1 cup milk
- 1/2 cup shredded cheese
- Salt and pepper to taste

Instructions:

1. Preheat the oven to 350°F (175°C).
2. In a saucepan, make a roux by cooking the flour with a bit of butter or oil for 1 minute over medium heat.
3. Gradually add the milk to the roux, stirring continuously until the mixture thickens.
4. Add the cheese to the saucepan and stir until melted and smooth.
5. Combine the cooked rice with the cheese sauce and season with salt and pepper.
6. Transfer the mixture to a baking dish and bake for 20 minutes until heated through.
7. Serve warm, checking that the rice and cheese bake is soft, moist, and easily spoonable to comply with Dysphagia Level 4 standards.

Nutritional Data:

Calories: 300 | Protein: 12g | Carbohydrates: 40g | Fat: 10g | Fiber: 1g | Sugar: 5g

112. Velvet Zucchini Blend

Preparation Time: 10 minutes | Cooking Time: 15 minutes

Ingredients:

- 1 large zucchini, peeled and chopped
- 2 tablespoons olive oil
- 1/4 cup low-sodium vegetable broth
- Salt to taste
- A pinch of ground nutmeg

Instructions:

1. In a medium saucepan, heat the olive oil over medium heat. Add the chopped zucchini and cook until tender, about 10-12 minutes.
2. Add the cooked zucchini and vegetable broth to a blender. Blend until smooth. If the mixture is too thick, add a little more broth to achieve a velvet-like consistency.
3. Add salt and a pinch of nutmeg (if using). Blend again to mix the seasonings evenly.
4. Serve warm. Ensure the blend is smooth and without lumps, suitable for Level 4 dysphagia requirements.

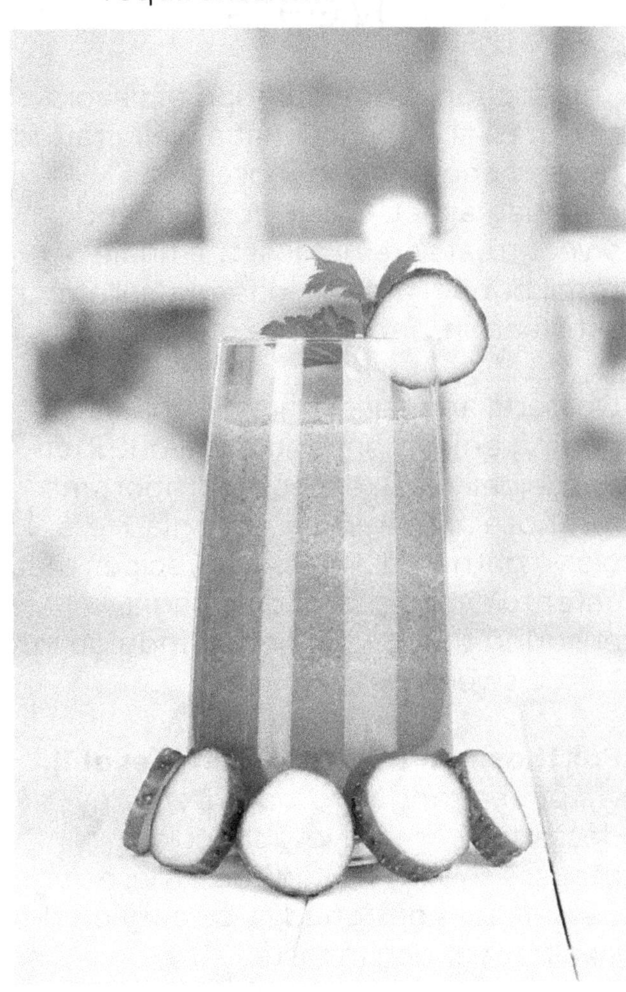

Nutritional Data:

Calories: 300 | Protein: 12g | Carbohydrates: 33g | Fat: 14g | Fiber: 2g | Sugar: 6g

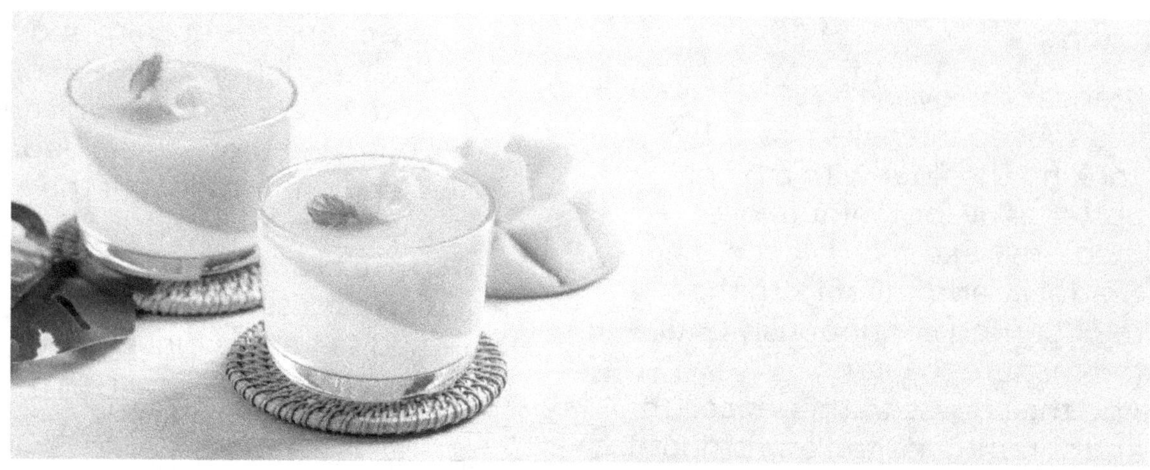

Desserts and Sweet Treats

This section is a celebration of flavors, textures, and the joy that a well-crafted dessert can bring to those on a dysphagia diet. Often, desserts and sweet treats are not just the finale of a meal but a highlight, offering comfort, satisfaction, and a sense of normalcy.

Desserts and snacks are essential for adding enjoyment and extra nutrition to the daily diet, especially important for those managing dysphagia. Here, we've gathered a variety of recipes that cater to every level of dysphagia, ensuring that everyone can indulge in a little sweetness.

For those on a Pureed Diet (Level 1), we offer a range of smooth, creamy desserts. From velvety chocolate mousse to silky fruit purees, these desserts are designed to be easy on the swallow yet rich in taste.

At the Soft and Well-Cooked level (Level 2), textures become more varied, including soft, moist cakes and tender baked fruits that provide a bit more substance while still being gentle and easy to consume.

Advancing to the Advanced Textures (Level 3), you'll find desserts that are closer to traditional favorites, like soft custards with ripe fruit toppings and moist, spongy cakes, all adapted to be safe and enjoyable.

For those following the Regular Diet with Modifications (Level 4), the selection expands to include a broader variety of sweet treats. Think of soft, chewy cookies, and modified pastries, prepared in ways that consider the dysphagia diet requirements.

Each recipe in this chapter is an invitation to indulge in the pleasures of dessert, reminding us that a dysphagia diet can still encompass the delights of sweet, tempting treats. We aim to make every spoonful or bite a delightful experience, ensuring that those with swallowing difficulties can still enjoy the pleasures of dessert.

Let's dive into a world where every dessert and treat is not only a delicious indulgence but also a safe and satisfying conclusion (or interlude) to any meal. With the "Dysphagia Cookbook," the joy of dessert remains an attainable and delightful part of the dietary journey.

LEVEL 1 RECIPES

113. Silky Mango Mousse

Preparation Time: 15 minutes | Cooking Time: 0 minutes (plus chilling time)

Ingredients:

- 1 ripe mango, peeled and stone removed
- 1 tbsp sugar or honey
- 1/2 cup whipped cream

Instructions:

1. Puree the mango in a blender until completely smooth.
2. Add sugar or honey to the mango puree and blend again to combine.
3. Gently fold the whipped cream into the mango puree to keep the mixture light and fluffy.
4. Spoon the mousse into a serving dish or individual cups.
5. Refrigerate for at least 1 hour to set.
6. Before serving, ensure the mousse maintains a smooth consistency that meets Dysphagia Level 1 standards.

Nutritional Data:
Calories: 200 | Protein: 1g | Carbohydrates: 30g | Fat: 10g | Fiber: 2g | Sugar: 28g

114. Creamy Vanilla Pudding

Preparation Time: 5 minutes | Cooking Time: 10 minutes (plus chilling time)

Ingredients:

- 1 cup milk
- 2 tbsp sugar
- 1 tsp vanilla extract
- 2 tbsp cornstarch

Instructions:

1. In a saucepan, combine the milk, sugar, and cornstarch. Cook over medium heat, stirring constantly, until the mixture thickens.
2. Once thickened, remove from heat and stir in the vanilla extract.
3. Pour the pudding into a serving dish or individual cups.
4. Refrigerate until set, usually about 1-2 hours.
5. Before serving, check the consistency to ensure that the pudding is smooth and creamy, appropriate for Dysphagia Level 1.

Nutritional Data:
Calories: 180 | Protein: 4g | Carbohydrates: 30g | Fat: 4g | Fiber: 0g | Sugar: 20g

115. Velvety Chocolate Avocado Pudding

Preparation Time: 10 minutes | Cooking Time: 0 minutes (plus chilling time)

Ingredients:

- 1 ripe avocado
- 2 tbsp cocoa powder
- 2 tbsp honey or maple syrup

Instructions:

1. Cut the avocado in half, remove the pit, and scoop the flesh into a blender.
2. Add the cocoa powder and honey or maple syrup to the avocado.
3. Blend until the mixture is completely smooth, without any lumps.

4. Taste and adjust the sweetness if needed.
5. Refrigerate the pudding for at least 1 hour to chill and set.
6. Before serving, stir the pudding to ensure it has a uniform, velvety consistency that meets Dysphagia Level 1 standards.

Nutritional Data:
Calories: 300 | Protein: 4g | Carbohydrates: 35g | Fat: 18g | Fiber: 10g | Sugar: 20g

116. Smooth Berry Gelatin

Preparation Time: 5 minutes | Cooking Time: 5 minutes (plus setting and blending time)

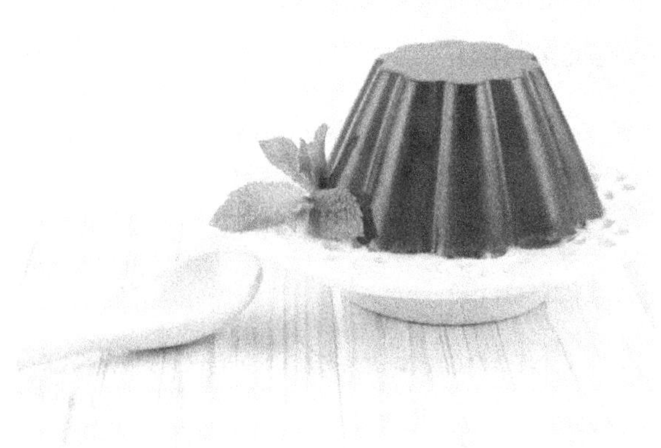

Ingredients:

- 1 package of berry-flavored gelatin
- 1 cup hot water
- 1/2 cup cold water
- 1/2 cup mixed berry puree

Instructions:

1. Dissolve the gelatin in hot water according to the package instructions.
2. Stir in the cold water and mix the berry puree.
3. Pour into a shallow dish and refrigerate until fully set, usually 2-3 hours.
4. Once set, blend the gelatin in a blender until it becomes smooth.
5. Serve chilled, ensuring the gelatin maintains a smooth, consistent texture appropriate for Dysphagia Level 1.

Nutritional Data:
Calories: 100 | Protein: 2g | Carbohydrates: 20g | Fat: 0g | Fiber: 1g | Sugar: 18g

117. Pumpkin Spice Puree

Preparation Time: 5 minutes | Cooking Time: 0 minutes

Ingredients:

- 1 cup pumpkin puree (not pumpkin pie filling)
- 1/4 tsp cinnamon
- A pinch of nutmeg
- A pinch of ginger
- 1 tbsp brown sugar

Instructions:

1. In a bowl, combine the pumpkin puree with cinnamon, nutmeg, ginger, and brown sugar.
2. Mix well until all the spices are thoroughly incorporated into the pumpkin.

3. For a smoother texture, blend the mixture until it achieves a uniform puree.
4. Taste and adjust the sweetness or spices if needed.
5. Serve the pumpkin spice puree at room temperature or chilled, ensuring it's smooth for Dysphagia Level 1 compliance.

Nutritional Data:
Calories: 120 | Protein: 2g | Carbohydrates: 30g | Fat: 0.5g | Fiber: 7g | Sugar: 13g

118. Silken Rice Pudding

Preparation Time: 5 minutes | Cooking Time: 25 minutes (plus blending time)

Ingredients:

- 1/2 cup cooked rice
- 1 cup milk
- 2 tbsp sugar
- 1/2 tsp vanilla extract

Instructions:

1. In a saucepan, combine cooked rice, milk, and sugar.
2. Cook over medium heat, stirring constantly until the mixture is creamy and the rice is completely soft, about 25 minutes.
3. Remove from heat and stir in the vanilla extract.
4. Allow the pudding to cool for a few minutes, then blend until completely smooth.
5. Serve the rice pudding at room temperature or chilled, ensuring it's perfectly smooth and spoonable for Dysphagia Level 1 compliance.

Nutritional Data:
Calories: 220 | Protein: 5g | Carbohydrates: 42g | Fat: 3g | Fiber: 0.5g | Sugar: 18g

119. Pureed Baked Apple with Cinnamon

Preparation Time: 10 minutes | Cooking Time: 30 minutes

Ingredients:

- 1 large apple, peeled and cored
- 1/2 tsp cinnamon
- 1 tbsp sugar
- 1/4 cup water

Instructions:

1. Preheat the oven to 350°F (175°C).
2. Cut the apples into cubes and place them in a small baking dish.
3. Sprinkle with cinnamon and sugar, then add water to the dish.
4. Cover with foil and bake until the apple cubes are very soft about 30 minutes.
5. Allow the apples to cool slightly, then transfer to a blender.
6. Puree the baked apple until smooth, adding a bit of water if needed to achieve a silky consistency.
7. Serve warm or chilled, ensuring the puree is smooth for Dysphagia Level 1 compliance.

Nutritional Data:
Calories: 90 | Protein: 0.5g | Carbohydrates: 24g | Fat: 0.2g | Fiber: 4g | Sugar: 19g

LEVEL2 RECIPES

120. Soft Baked Custard

Preparation Time: 10 minutes | Cooking Time: 35 minutes

Ingredients:

- 2 eggs
- 1 cup milk
- 2 tbsp sugar
- 1/2 tsp vanilla extract

Instructions:

1. Preheat the oven to 325°F (165°C).
2. In a bowl, whisk together eggs, milk, sugar, and vanilla extract until well combined.
3. Pour the mixture into a small baking dish or ramekin.
4. Place the dish in a larger baking pan and fill the pan with hot water to about halfway up the side of the custard dish (water bath).
5. Bake until the custard is set but still quivering in the center, about 35 minutes.
6. Remove from the oven and water bath, and let cool slightly. The custard should be soft and smooth, fitting for Dysphagia Level 2 compliance.
7. Serve the custard warm or chilled, as preferred.

Nutritional Data:
Calories: 180 | Protein: 9g | Carbohydrates: 20g | Fat: 7g | Fiber: 0g | Sugar: 20g

121. Creamy Banana Yogurt Parfait

Preparation Time: 5 minutes | Cooking Time: 0 minutes

Ingredients:

- 1 cup plain or vanilla yogurt
- 1 ripe banana
- Optional honey or maple syrup for sweetness

Instructions:

1. Slice the banana into soft, thin pieces.
2. In a serving glass or bowl, begin with a layer of yogurt.
3. Add a layer of banana slices on top of the yogurt.
4. Drizzle a small amount of honey or maple syrup over the bananas if desired.
5. Repeat the layers until all ingredients are used.
6. Serve immediately, ensuring the banana slices are soft and the yogurt is creamy for Dysphagia Level 2 compliance.

Nutritional Data:
Calories: 220 | Protein: 8g | Carbohydrates: 42g | Fat: 3g | Fiber: 2g | Sugar: 30g (varies if sweetener is added)

122. Tender Stewed Fruit Compote

Preparation Time: 10 minutes | Cooking Time: 30 minutes

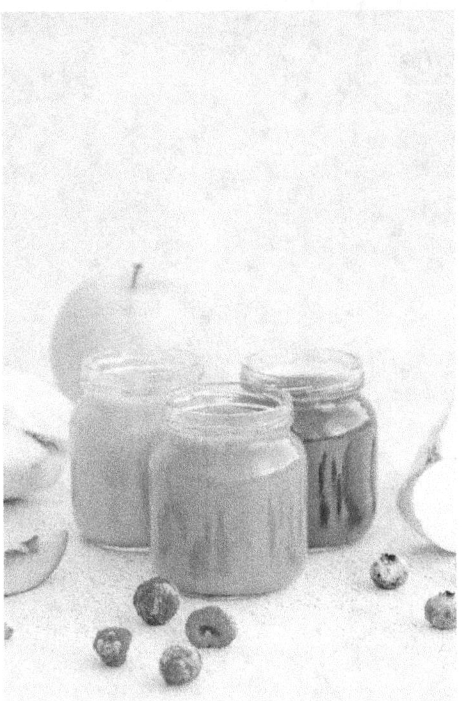

Ingredients:

- 1 apple, peeled and diced
- 1 pear, peeled and diced
- 1 peach, peeled and diced
- 2 tbsp sugar
- 1/2 tsp cinnamon
- Water to cover

Instructions:

1. Combine the diced fruits, sugar, cinnamon, and enough water to cover the fruits in a saucepan.
2. Cook over medium heat until the fruits are soft and the liquid has reduced to a syrupy consistency, about 30 minutes.
3. Mash the fruits gently to ensure they are soft enough while still retaining some texture.
4. Serve warm or chilled, checking that the compote is tender for Dysphagia Level 2 compliance.

Nutritional Data:
Calories: 180 | Protein: 1g | Carbohydrates: 46g | Fat: 0.5g | Fiber: 5g | Sugar: 40g

123. Moist Carrot Cake Pudding

Preparation Time: 5 minutes | Cooking Time: 0 minutes (assuming carrot cake is pre-baked)

Ingredients:

- 1 slice soft-baked carrot cake
- 1/4 cup milk or cream

Instructions:

1. Crumble the carrot cake into a bowl.
2. Pour milk or cream over the crumbled cake.
3. Use a hand blender or food processor to blend the mixture until it has a smooth, pudding-like consistency.
4. Adjust the amount of milk or cream if necessary to achieve the desired texture.
5. Serve immediately, ensuring the pudding is soft and moist, suitable for Dysphagia Level 2 compliance.

Nutritional Data:
Calories: Approximately 300 (varies based on the size of the cake slice and type of milk or cream) | Protein: 4g | Carbohydrates: 45g | Fat: 12g | Fiber: 1g | Sugar: 30g

124. Soft Poached Pears in Vanilla Syrup

Preparation Time: 5 minutes | Cooking Time: 20 minutes

Ingredients:

- 1 large pear, peeled and cored
- 2 tbsp sugar
- 1 tsp vanilla extract
- Enough water to cover the pears in the pan

Instructions:

1. Cut the pear into slices or cubes, depending on preference.
2. In a saucepan, combine water, sugar, and vanilla extract, and bring to a simmer.
3. Add the pear slices or cubes to the pan and simmer gently until they are tender about 20 minutes.
4. Once the pears are soft, remove them from heat and let them cool slightly.
5. Serve the pears with a bit of the vanilla syrup, ensuring they are soft and moist, compliant with Dysphagia Level 2 standards.

Nutritional Data:
Calories: 150 | Protein: 0.5g | Carbohydrates: 38g | Fat: 0.2g | Fiber: 4g | Sugar: 33g

125. Mango and Coconut Rice Pudding

Preparation Time: 10 minutes | Cooking Time: 30 minutes

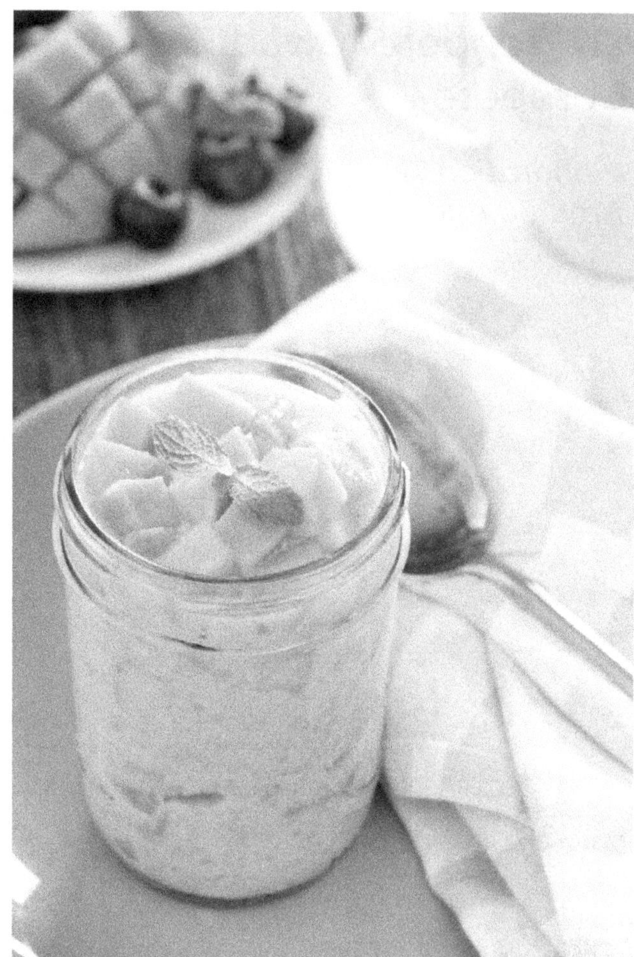

Ingredients:

- 1/2 cup Arborio rice (suitable for a soft, creamy texture)
- 2 cups coconut milk (for creaminess and flavor)
- 1/4 cup sugar (adjust to taste)
- 1 ripe mango, pureed (for natural sweetness and flavor)
- 1/2 tsp vanilla extract
- A pinch of salt

Instructions:

1. Combine Arborio rice, coconut milk, and a pinch of salt in a saucepan. Bring to a simmer over medium heat, stirring occasionally.
2. Once simmering, reduce the heat to low and cook for about 25-30 minutes, or until the rice is very soft and the mixture has

thickened to a creamy consistency.

3. While the rice is cooking, puree the ripe mango in a blender until smooth.
4. When the rice is cooked, stir in the sugar and vanilla extract. Remove from heat.
5. Gently fold in the mango puree until well combined.
6. Serve the pudding warm or chilled, depending on preference.
7. Ensure the consistency is appropriate for Dysphagia Level 2. If necessary, blend the pudding to achieve a mildly thick, smooth consistency.

Nutritional Data:
Calories: 200 | Protein: 2g | Carbohydrates: 30g | Fat: 07g | Fiber: 2g | Sugar: 15g

126. Rice Pudding with Soft Raisins

Preparation Time: 5 minutes | Cooking Time: 25 minutes

Ingredients:

- 1/2 cup cooked white rice
- 1 cup milk
- 2 tbsp sugar
- 1/4 cup raisins
- 1/2 tsp vanilla extract

Instructions:

1. Combine the milk, cooked rice, and sugar in a saucepan over medium heat.
2. Cook while stirring frequently until the mixture thickens and the rice is completely soft, about 20 minutes.
3. Add the raisins and vanilla extract to the mixture and cook

for an additional 5 minutes, ensuring the raisins become plump and soft.
4. Allow the pudding to cool slightly, then serve warm, ensuring the raisins and rice are soft enough to meet Dysphagia Level 2 standards.

Nutritional Data:
Calories: 220 | Protein: 5g | Carbohydrates: 45g | Fat: 2g | Fiber: 1g | Sugar: 25g

LEVEL3 RECIPES

127. Soft-Baked Apple Crisp

Preparation Time: 10 minutes | Cooking Time: 30 minutes

Ingredients:

- 1 large apple, peeled and sliced
- 1/4 cup oatmeal
- 2 tbsp brown sugar
- 1 tbsp butter, melted
- 1/2 tsp cinnamon

Instructions:

1. Preheat the oven to 350°F (175°C).
2. Place the sliced apples in a small baking dish.
3. In a bowl, mix the oatmeal, brown sugar, melted butter, and cinnamon until it forms a soft crumble.
4. Spread the oatmeal mixture over the sliced apples.
5. Bake for 30 minutes, or until the apples are tender and the topping is soft but crumbly.
6. Allow the apple crisp to cool slightly to ensure it's at a safe temperature and the apples are

soft enough to meet Dysphagia Level 3 requirements.

7. Serve warm, checking the texture to make sure it can be chewed with minimal effort.

Nutritional Data:
Calories: 250 | Protein: 2g | Carbohydrates: 45g | Fat: 8g | Fiber: 4g | Sugar: 30g

128. Moist Lemon Sponge Cake

Preparation Time: 15 minutes | Cooking Time: 25 minutes

Ingredients:

- 1/2 cup flour
- 1/2 cup sugar
- 2 eggs
- Zest of 1 lemon
- 1 tsp baking powder

Instructions:

1. Preheat the oven to 350°F (175°C). Grease a small cake pan.
2. In a bowl, beat the eggs and sugar until light and fluffy.
3. Gently fold in the flour, lemon zest, and baking powder until just combined.
4. Pour the batter into the prepared pan.
5. Bake for 25 minutes, or until a toothpick inserted into the center comes out clean.
6. Allow the cake to cool, then cut into small, easy-to-chew pieces.
7. Ensure the sponge cake is moist and has a delicate crumb to comply with Dysphagia Level 3 standards before serving.

Nutritional Data:
Calories: 300 | Protein: 6g | Carbohydrates: 55g | Fat: 7g | Fiber: 1g | Sugar: 35g

129. Tender Blueberry Muffins

Preparation Time: 10 minutes | Cooking Time: 20 minutes

Ingredients:

- 1 cup flour
- 1/2 cup blueberries
- 1/4 cup sugar
- 1 egg
- 1/2 cup milk

Instructions:

1. Preheat the oven to 375°F (190°C) and grease a muffin tin.
2. In a bowl, mix the flour and sugar.
3. In another bowl, beat the egg and then add the milk.
4. Combine the wet and dry ingredients, stirring until just mixed.
5. Gently fold in the blueberries.
6. Spoon the batter into the muffin tin.
7. Bake for 20 minutes or until a toothpick comes out clean.
8. Let the muffins cool and check to ensure the blueberries are tender and the muffin is soft enough for Dysphagia Level 3 compliance before serving.

Nutritional Data:
Calories: 150 per muffin | Protein: 3g | Carbohydrates: 28g | Fat: 3g | Fiber: 1g | Sugar: 10g

130. Creamy Cheesecake with Soft Fruit Topping

Preparation Time: 15 minutes | Cooking Time: 45 minutes (plus chilling time)

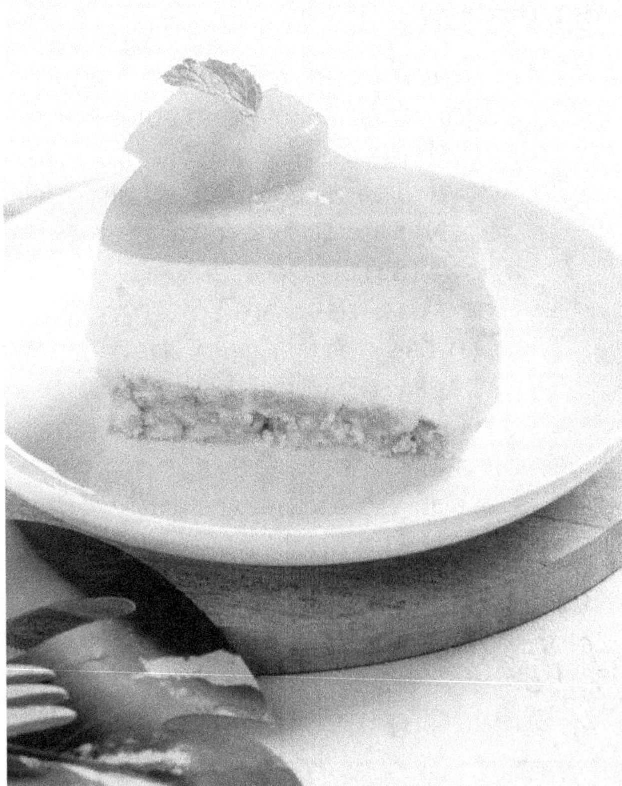

Ingredients:

- 1/2 cup cream cheese
- 2 tbsp sugar
- 1 egg
- 1/4 cup graham cracker crumbs
- 1/2 cup soft fruit compote

Instructions:

1. Preheat the oven to 325°F (163°C).
2. Mix the graham cracker crumbs with a little melted butter and press into the bottom of a small baking dish to form a crust.
3. In a bowl, beat the cream cheese and sugar until smooth.
4. Add the egg and beat until combined.
5. Pour the cream cheese mixture over the crust.
6. Bake for 45 minutes until the cheesecake is set but slightly jiggly in the center.
7. Allow to cool, then chill in the refrigerator for at least 4 hours.
8. Top with the soft fruit compote before serving, ensuring the fruit is tender and the cheesecake is soft enough for Dysphagia Level 3 compliance.

Nutritional Data:
Calories: 300 | Protein: 6g | Carbohydrates: 25g | Fat: 20g | Fiber: 1g | Sugar: 18g

131. Fluffy Chocolate Mousse

Preparation Time: 15 minutes | Cooking Time: 0 minutes (plus chilling time)

Ingredients:

- 2 oz chocolate
- 1 egg, separated
- 2 tbsp sugar
- 1/2 cup whipped cream

Instructions:

1. Melt the chocolate in a heatproof bowl over a pan of simmering water, then let it cool slightly.
2. In a separate bowl, whisk the egg white until stiff peaks form, gradually adding 1 tablespoon of sugar.
3. In another bowl, whisk the egg yolk with the remaining sugar until pale and creamy.
4. Fold the melted chocolate into the egg yolk mixture.

5. Gently fold in the whipped cream until fully incorporated, and then carefully fold in the egg white.
6. Spoon the mixture into a serving dish and chill in the refrigerator for at least 2 hours.
7. Before serving, check that the mousse maintains a light and smooth consistency suitable for Dysphagia Level 3 compliance.

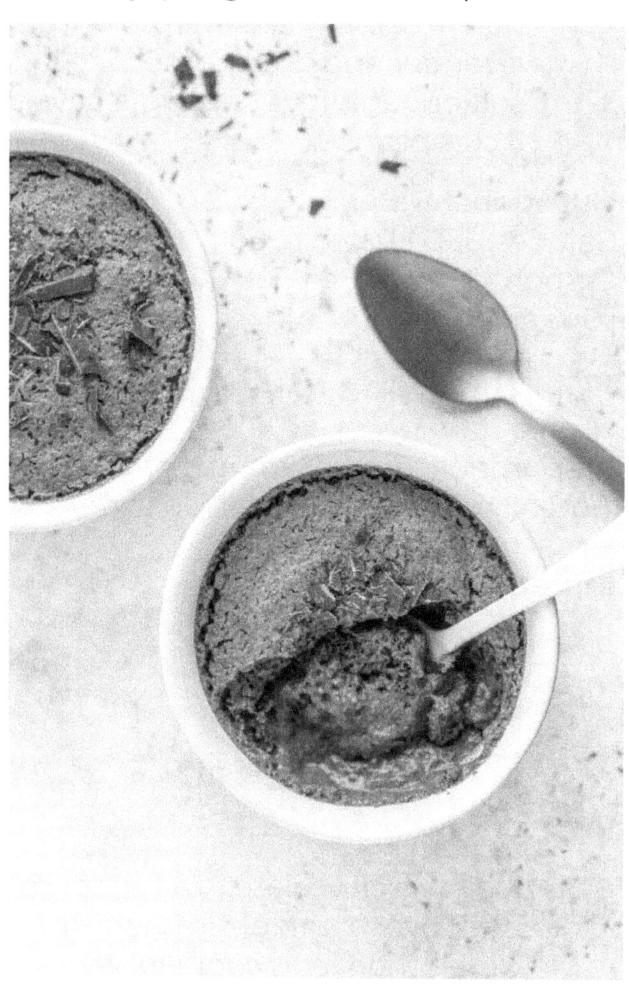

Nutritional Data:
Calories: 300 | Protein: 5g | Carbohydrates: 26g | Fat: 20g | Fiber: 1g | Sugar: 24g

132. Soft Poached Fruit Medley

Preparation Time: 10 minutes | Cooking Time: 15 minutes

Ingredients:

- 1 cup mixed fruits (like pears, peaches, and apricots), peeled and sliced
- 2 tbsp sugar
- 2 cups water
- 1/2 tsp vanilla extract or a pinch of cinnamon for flavor

Instructions:

1. In a saucepan, bring the water, sugar, and vanilla extract or cinnamon to a simmer.
2. Add the sliced fruits and simmer gently until they are tender about 15 minutes.
3. Once the fruits are soft, remove from the heat and let them cool in the syrup.
4. Serve the poached fruits with a bit of their syrup, ensuring they are soft enough to comply with Dysphagia Level 3 standards.

Nutritional Data:
Calories: 120 | Protein: 1g | Carbohydrates: 30g | Fat: 0.2g | Fiber: 3g | Sugar: 27g

133. Baked Rice Pudding with Soft Raisins

Preparation Time: 15 minutes | Cooking Time: 60 minutes

Ingredients:

- 1/4 cup rice
- 2 cups milk
- 1/4 cup sugar
- 1 egg
- 1/4 cup raisins
- 1/2 tsp vanilla extract

Instructions:

1. Preheat your oven to 325°F (163°C).
2. In a saucepan, combine the rice and milk. Bring to a simmer and cook over low heat for 20 minutes, stirring occasionally.
3. In a separate bowl, whisk the egg and sugar together until well combined.
4. Temper the egg mixture by adding a small amount of the hot rice mixture while continuously whisking to prevent curdling.
5. Pour the tempered egg mixture back into the saucepan with the rice and milk, and cook for an additional 5 minutes, stirring constantly.
6. Stir in the raisins and vanilla extract.
7. Transfer the mixture to a greased baking dish and bake for 30-35 minutes, or until the pudding is set but still soft.
8. Let it cool slightly before serving to ensure it's suitable for Dysphagia Level 3.

Nutritional Data:
Calories: 300 | Protein: 7g | Carbohydrates: 57g | Fat: 6g | Fiber: 1g | Sugar: 35g

LEVEL4 RECIPES

134. Soft-Baked Peach Cobbler

Preparation Time: 20 minutes | Cooking Time: 30 minutes

Ingredients:

- 2 cups peaches, peeled and sliced
- 1/2 cup flour
- 1/4 cup sugar
- 2 tbsp butter
- 1/2 tsp baking powder

Instructions:

1. Preheat your oven to 350°F (177°C).
2. In a mixing bowl, combine the flour, sugar, and baking powder.
3. Cut in the butter until the mixture resembles coarse crumbs.
4. Place the sliced peaches in a greased baking dish.
5. Sprinkle the flour mixture over the peaches.
6. Bake for 30 minutes, or until the topping is golden brown and the peaches are soft.
7. Allow it to cool slightly before serving to ensure it's suitable for Dysphagia Level 4.

Nutritional Data:
Calories: 230 | Protein: 2g | Carbohydrates: 47g | Fat: 5g | Fiber: 2g | Sugar: 29g

135. Creamy Banana Bread

Preparation Time: 15 minutes | Cooking Time: 60 minutes

Ingredients:

- 2 ripe bananas, mashed
- 1 1/2 cups flour
- 1 cup sugar
- 2 eggs
- 1 tsp baking soda

Instructions:

1. Preheat your oven to 350°F (177°C) and grease a loaf pan.
2. In a mixing bowl, combine the mashed bananas, sugar, and eggs. Mix until well combined.

3. Add the flour and baking soda to the banana mixture and stir until the batter is smooth.
4. Pour the batter into the greased loaf pan.
5. Bake for 60 minutes, or until a toothpick inserted into the center comes out clean.
6. Allow the banana bread to cool slightly before serving to ensure it's suitable for Dysphagia Level 4

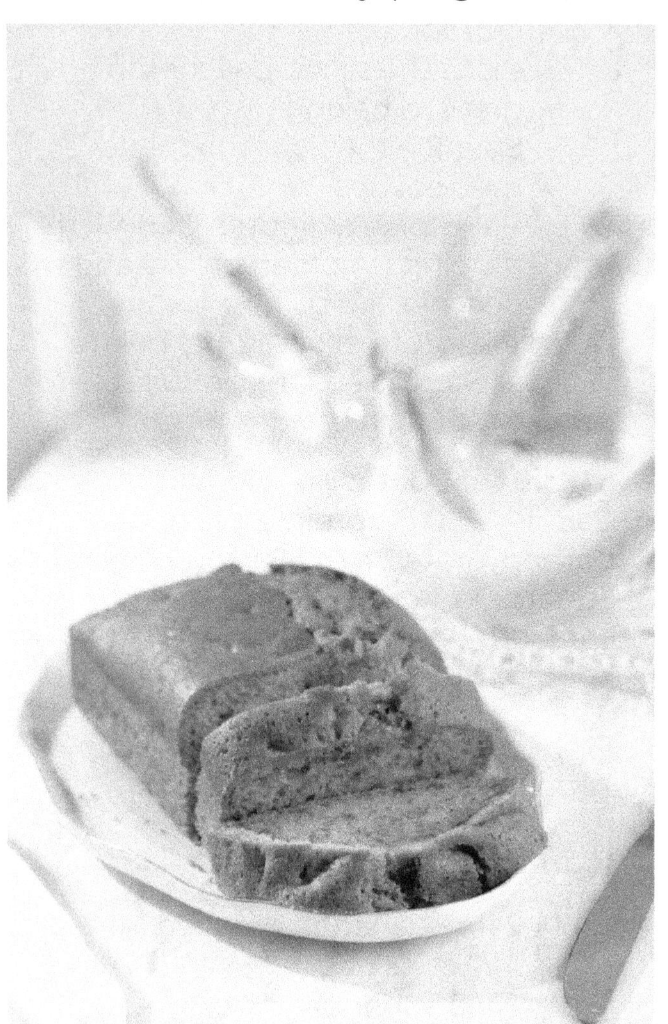

Nutritional Data:
Calories: 180 | Protein: 3g |
Carbohydrates: 37g | Fat: 2g | Fiber: 1g |
Sugar: 20g

136. Tender Fruit Trifle

*Preparation Time: 30 minutes |
Cooking Time: 0 minutes*

Ingredients:

- 1 cup sponge cake, cut into small pieces
- 1 cup vanilla custard
- 1/2 cup whipped cream
- 1/2 cup soft fruits (e.g., berries or banana), diced

Instructions:

1. In a serving glass or bowl, place a layer of sponge cake pieces.
2. Add a layer of diced soft fruits on top of the cake.
3. Pour a layer of vanilla custard over the fruits.
4. Repeat the layers until the glass or bowl is filled.
5. Top with a dollop of whipped cream.
6. Serve immediately.

Nutritional Data:
Calories: 300 | Protein: 3g |
Carbohydrates: 45g | Fat: 12g | Fiber: 2g
| Sugar: 25g

137. Fluffy Angel Food Cake with Soft Berry Compote

Preparation Time: 20 minutes | Cooking Time: 45 minutes

Ingredients:

- 4 egg whites
- 1 cup sugar
- 1 cup flour
- Mixed berries (e.g., strawberries, blueberries, raspberries) for compote

Instructions:

1. Preheat your oven to 350°F (177°C).
2. In a mixing bowl, beat the egg whites until stiff peaks form.
3. Gradually add the sugar while continuing to beat the egg whites.
4. Gently fold in the flour, being careful not to deflate the egg whites.
5. Pour the batter into an ungreased cake pan.
6. Bake for 45 minutes or until the cake is golden brown and springs back when touched.
7. While the cake is cooling, gently cook the mixed berries in a saucepan until they become soft.
8. Serve the fluffy angel food cake with a side of the soft berry compote.

Nutritional Data:
Calories: 150 | Protein: 3g | Carbohydrates: 34g | Fat: 0g | Fiber: 2g | Sugar: 18g

138. Moist Carrot Cake with Cream Cheese Frosting

Preparation Time: 20 minutes | Cooking Time: 35 minutes

Ingredients

- 1 cup grated carrots
- 1 cup flour
- 1 cup sugar
- 2 eggs
- 1 tsp cinnamon
- Cream cheese for frosting

Instructions:

1. Preheat your oven to 350°F (177°C) and grease a cake pan.
2. In a mixing bowl, combine the grated carrots, sugar, and eggs. Mix until well combined.
3. Add the flour and cinnamon to the carrot mixture and stir until the batter is smooth.
4. Pour the batter into the greased cake pan.
5. Bake for 35 minutes, or until a toothpick inserted into the center comes out clean.
6. Allow the carrot cake to cool, then frost it with cream cheese.

Nutritional Data:
Calories: 220 | Protein: 4g | Carbohydrates: 43g | Fat: 4g | Fiber: 1g | Sugar: 25g

139. Soft Pumpkin Pie

Preparation Time: 20 minutes | Cooking Time: 45 minutes

Ingredients:

- 1 cup pumpkin puree
- 2 eggs
- 1/2 cup sugar
- 1 tsp cinnamon
- 1/2 tsp ginger
- Pie crust

Instructions:

1. Preheat your oven to 375°F (190°C).
2. In a mixing bowl, combine the pumpkin puree, eggs, sugar, cinnamon, and ginger. Mix until well combined.
3. Line a pie pan with the pie crust.
4. Pour the pumpkin mixture into the pie crust.
5. Bake for 45 minutes or until the filling is set.
6. Allow the pumpkin pie to cool before serving.

Nutritional Data:
Calories: 220 | Protein: 4g | Carbohydrates: 33g | Fat: 8g | Fiber: 2g | Sugar: 17g

140. Creamy Chocolate Pudding

Preparation Time: 10 minutes | Cooking Time: 15 minutes

Ingredients:

- 2 cups milk
- 1/2 cup sugar
- 1/4 cup cocoa powder
- 3 tbsp cornstarch

Instructions:

1. In a saucepan, combine the sugar, cocoa powder, and cornstarch.
2. Gradually whisk in the milk until the mixture is smooth.
3. Place the saucepan over medium heat and cook, stirring constantly, until the pudding thickens (about 10-15 minutes).
4. Remove from heat and let it cool before serving.

Nutritional Data:
Calories: 150 | Protein: 3g | Carbohydrates: 32g | Fat: 3g | Fiber: 2g | Sugar: 20g

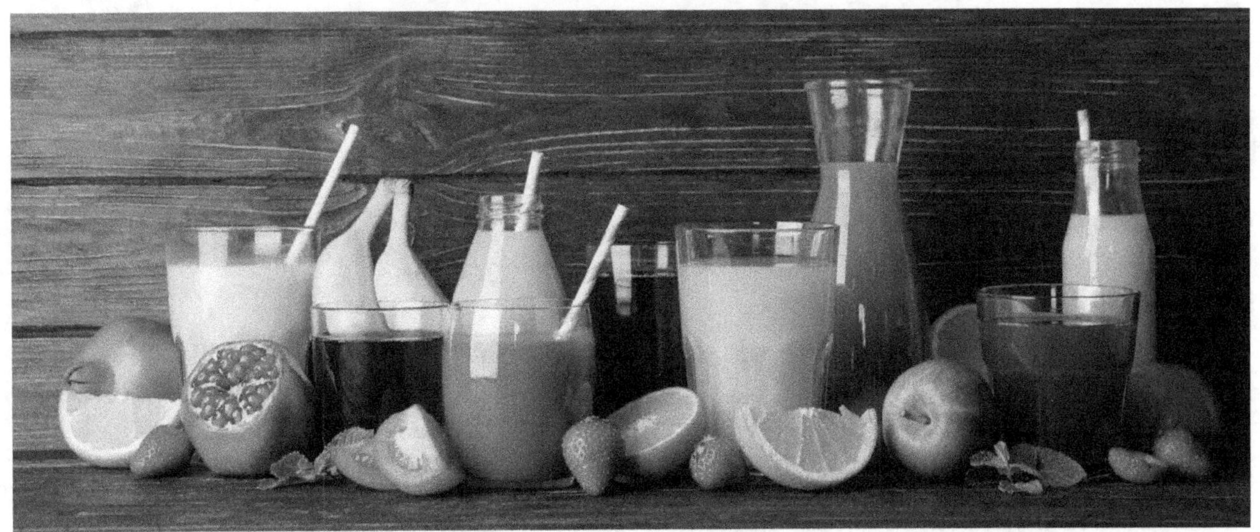

Beverages and Smoothies

This section is all about quenching thirst and providing nutritional boosts in the most delightful way for those with dysphagia. Understanding the importance of hydration and the challenges that swallowing difficulties can present, we have tailored a variety of drink options to suit various needs and preferences.

Beverages and smoothies are not only vital for hydration but also offer an opportunity to incorporate a wide range of vitamins, minerals, and other nutrients in an easily consumable form. In this chapter, you'll find an array of recipes, from thickened drinks to nutrient-packed smoothies, each designed to be both safe to swallow and a pleasure to sip.

For individuals following a Pureed Diet (Level 1), the focus is on thickened beverages and smoothies that are smooth and free from lumps. These drinks are carefully thickened to the right consistency, ensuring safe swallowing. Recipes include everything from thickened fruit juices to creamy, blended smoothies enriched with yogurt or protein powder.

Moving to the Soft and Well-Cooked level (Level 2), we introduce beverages with a little more texture, such as smoothies with finely blended soft fruits and vegetable juices. These are ideal for those who can handle some texture but still need their drinks to be relatively smooth and easy to swallow.

In the Advanced Textures (Level 3) category, the drinks become less restricted, allowing for more variety in ingredients. These beverages might include softer chunks or bits, suitable for those who can manage more texture. Think of smoothies with small, soft fruit pieces or lightly textured milkshakes.

For those on the Regular Diet with Modifications (Level 4), the beverages and smoothies can include an even broader range of ingredients, though still avoiding extremely hard, sticky, or chewy additives. This level offers more traditional beverage options, modified as necessary to ensure they are still safe and enjoyable to consume.

LEVEL 1 RECIPES

141. Thickened Apple Juice

Preparation Time: 5 minutes

Ingredients:

- 1 cup apple juice
- Commercial thickening agent

Instructions:

1. Pour the apple juice into a glass.
2. Add the commercial thickening agent to the juice.
3. Stir until the juice reaches a nectar-like consistency.

Nutritional Data:
Calories: 60 | Carbohydrates: 15g | Sugar: 12g

142. Creamy Vanilla Thickened Milkshake

Preparation Time: 5 minutes

Ingredients:

- 1 cup milk
- 2 scoops vanilla ice cream
- Commercial thickening agent
- 1/2 tsp vanilla extract

Instructions:

1. In a blender, combine the milk, vanilla ice cream, and vanilla extract.
2. Add the commercial thickening agent to the mixture.
3. Blend until the milkshake reaches a thick and creamy consistency.
4. Pour into a glass and serve.

Nutritional Data:
Calories: 250 | Protein: 6g | Carbohydrates: 30g | Fat: 12g | Sugar: 26g

143. Smooth Berry Puree Smoothie

Preparation Time: 5 minutes

Ingredients:

- 1 cup mixed berries (strawberries, blueberries, raspberries)
- 2 tbsp yogurt
- Commercial thickening agent

Instructions:

1. Place the mixed berries in a blender.
2. Add the yogurt to the blender.
3. Sprinkle the commercial thickening agent over the ingredients.
4. Blend until the mixture reaches a smooth and thickened consistency.
5. Pour into a glass and serve.

Nutritional Data:
Calories: 90 | Carbohydrates: 20g | Fiber: 5g | Sugar: 12g

144. Velvety Chocolate Thickened Beverage

Preparation Time: 5 minutes

Ingredients:

- 1 cup milk
- 2 tbsp cocoa powder
- 2 tbsp sugar
- Commercial thickening agent

Instructions:

1. In a saucepan, heat the milk over low heat.
2. Stir in the cocoa powder and sugar until well combined.
3. Add the commercial thickening agent to the mixture.
4. Cook and stir until the beverage thickens to the desired consistency.
5. Pour into a mug and serve.

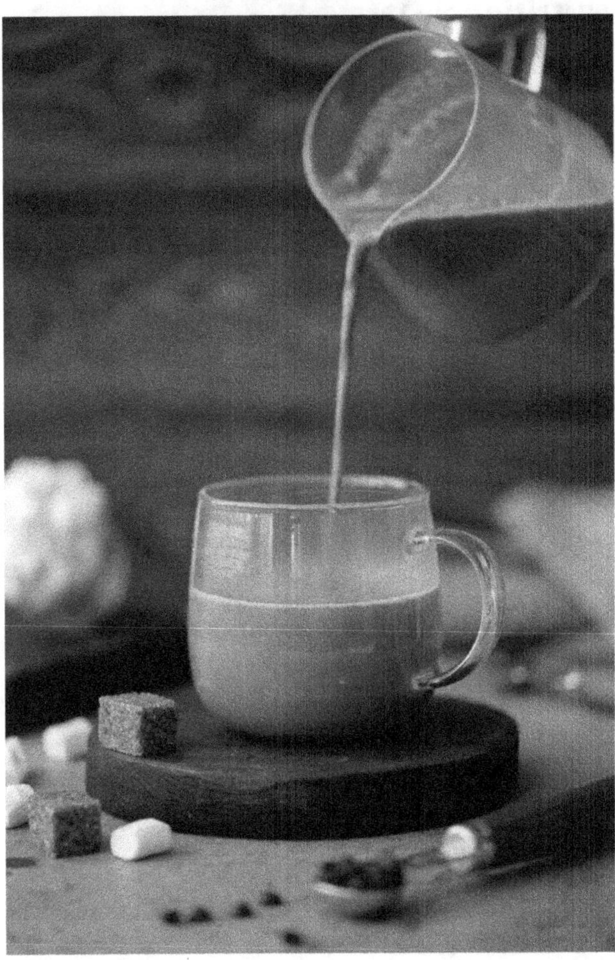

Nutritional Data:
Calories: 180 | Protein: 7g | Carbohydrates: 30g | Fat: 5g | Sugar: 24g

145. Thickened Mango Nectar

Preparation Time: 5 minutes

Ingredients:

- 1 cup mango nectar or pureed mango
- Commercial thickening agent

Instructions:

1. Place the mango nectar or pureed mango in a container.
2. Sprinkle the commercial thickening agent over the mango.
3. Stir well until the nectar reaches a thickened and safe-to-swallow consistency.
4. Pour into a glass and serve.

Nutritional Data:
Calories: 120 | Carbohydrates: 30g | Fiber: 2g | Sugar: 28g

LEVEL2 RECIPES

146. Creamy Banana Smoothie

Preparation Time: 5 minutes

Ingredients:

- 1 ripe banana
- 1 cup milk or yogurt
- A small amount of thickening agent

Instructions:

1. Peel the ripe banana and place it in a blender.
2. Add the milk or yogurt to the blender.
3. Sprinkle a small amount of thickening agent over the ingredients.
4. Blend until smooth and creamy.
5. Pour into a glass and serve.

Nutritional Data:
Calories: 180 | Carbohydrates: 36g |
Protein: 6g | Fat: 2g | Fiber: 3g | Sugar:
22g

147. Soft Berry Yogurt Drink

Preparation Time: 5 minutes

Ingredients:

- Mixed berries (like strawberries and blueberries)
- Plain or vanilla yogurt

Instructions:

1. Place the mixed berries in a blender.
2. Add plain or vanilla yogurt to the blender.
3. Blend until the mixture reaches a smooth and soft texture.
4. Pour into a glass and serve.

Nutritional Data:
Calories: 150 | Carbohydrates: 30g |
Protein: 6g | Fat: 2g | Fiber: 5g | Sugar:
20g

148. Gentle Peach and Pear Nectar

Preparation Time: 10 minutes

Ingredients:

- Ripe peaches
- Ripe pears
- Water or apple juice
- Optional thickening agent

Instructions:

1. Wash, peel, and remove the pits from the ripe peaches and pears.
2. Cut the peaches and pears into small, manageable pieces.
3. Place the fruit pieces in a blender.
4. Add a small amount of water or apple juice to help with blending.
5. If needed, include the optional thickening agent for a slightly thicker consistency.
6. Blend until the mixture becomes smooth and reaches the desired thickness.
7. Pour into a glass and serve.

Nutritional Data:
Calories: 120 | Carbohydrates: 30g |
Protein: 2g | Fat: 0.5g | Fiber: 5g | Sugar:
20g

149. Smooth Avocado and Honey Shake

Preparation Time: 5 minutes

Ingredients:

- Ripe avocado
- Milk or almond milk
- Honey
- Optional thickening agent

Instructions:

1. Cut the ripe avocado in half and remove the pit.
2. Scoop out the avocado flesh and place it in a blender.
3. Add milk or almond milk to the blender.
4. Include honey for sweetness, and adjust the amount to your preference.
5. If needed, add the optional thickening agent.
6. Blend until the mixture is smooth and reaches a soft, drinkable texture.
7. Pour into a glass and serve.

LEVEL3 RECIPES

150. Tender Peach Smoothie

Preparation Time: 5 minutes

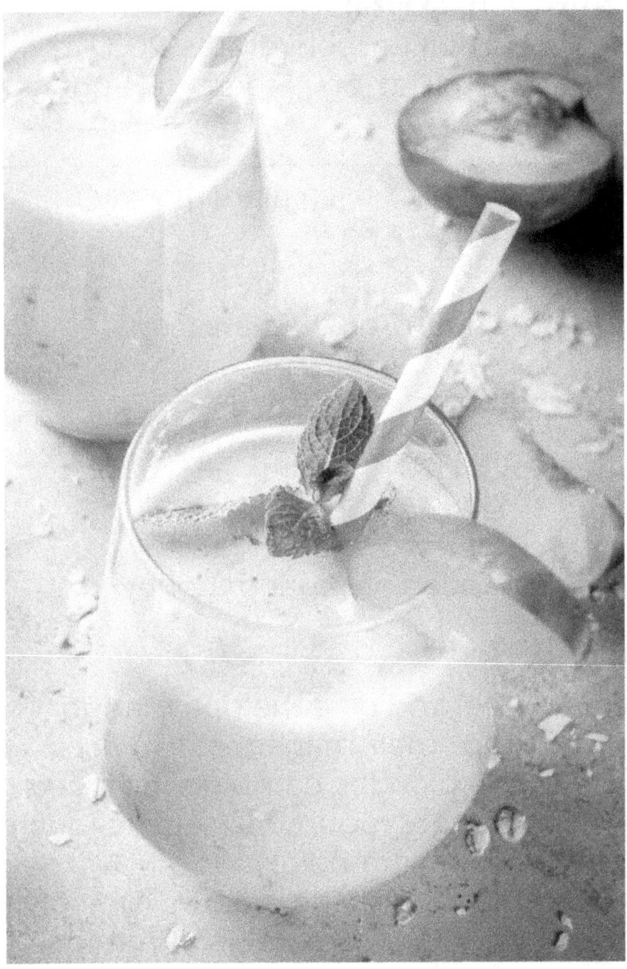

Ingredients:

- Ripe peaches
- Yogurt or milk
- Honey (optional)

Instructions:

1. Wash, peel, and remove the pits from the ripe peaches.
2. Cut the peaches into small, manageable pieces.
3. Place the peach pieces in a blender.
4. Add yogurt or milk to the blender.
5. Include honey for sweetness, and adjust the amount to your preference.
6. Blend until the mixture is smooth with small, manageable fruit pieces.
7. Pour into a glass and serve.

Nutritional Data:
Calories: 150 | Carbohydrates: 30g |
Protein: 4g | Fat: 2g | Fiber: 3g | Sugar:
27g

151. Soft Mixed Berry Compote Drink

Preparation Time: 10 minutes

Ingredients:

- Mixed berries (like strawberries, blueberries, raspberries)
- Water
- Sugar or honey

Instructions:

1. Wash the mixed berries and place them in a blender.
2. Add water to the blender.
3. Include sugar or honey for sweetness, and adjust the amount to your preference.
4. Blend until the mixture is lightly textured, with small, soft fruit pieces remaining for a bit of texture.
5. Pour into a glass and serve.

Nutritional Data:
Calories: 80 | Carbohydrates: 20g |
Protein: 1g | Fat: 0g | Fiber: 4g | Sugar:
16g

152. Creamy Oatmeal and Banana Shake

Preparation Time: 15 minutes

Ingredients:

- Cooked oatmeal
- Ripe banana
- Milk
- Cinnamon

Instructions:

1. Cook oatmeal according to package instructions and let it cool to room temperature.
2. Peel the ripe banana and cut it into small pieces.
3. Place cooked oatmeal, banana pieces, milk, and a pinch of cinnamon in a blender.
4. Blend until the mixture is soft but slightly textured in consistency.
5. Pour into a glass and serve.

Nutritional Data:
Calories: 200 | Carbohydrates: 45g | Protein: 6g | Fat: 2g | Fiber: 6g | Sugar: 15g

153. Soft Apple and Cinnamon Swirl

Preparation Time: 10 minutes

Ingredients:

- Apple puree
- Water or apple juice
- Cinnamon
- Nutmeg

Instructions:

1. In a saucepan, combine apple puree and water or apple juice.
2. Add cinnamon and nutmeg for flavor.
3. Heat the mixture over low heat, stirring continuously until warm and well combined.
4. Pour into a mug or glass and serve as a warm, apple-cinnamon-flavored drink with a pureed apple base and a swirl of soft texture.

Nutritional Data:
Calories: 80 | Carbohydrates: 20g | Protein: 1g | Fat: 0g | Fiber: 4g | Sugar: 16g

154. Mildly Chunky Mango Lassi

Preparation Time: 10 minutes

Ingredients:

- Ripe mango
- Yogurt
- Milk
- A touch of sugar or honey

Instructions:

1. Peel and dice the ripe mango into small, manageable pieces.
2. In a blender, combine the diced mango, yogurt, milk, and a touch of sugar or honey.
3. Blend until the mixture is mildly chunky with small, soft mango pieces.
4. Pour into a glass and serve as a traditional mango lassi with a gentle texture.

Nutritional Data:
Calories: 180 | Carbohydrates: 40g | Protein: 5g | Fat: 2g | Fiber: 4g | Sugar: 36g

LEVEL4 RECIPES

155. Gentle Pear and Ginger Smoothie

Preparation Time: 10 minutes

Ingredients:

- Ripe pears
- A small piece of fresh ginger
- Yogurt or milk
- Honey (optional)

Instructions:

1. Peel and dice the ripe pears into small, manageable pieces.
2. Peel and chop a small piece of fresh ginger.
3. In a blender, combine the diced pears, chopped ginger, yogurt or milk, and honey if desired.
4. Blend until the mixture is pureed to a soft consistency with small, manageable fruit pieces for texture.
5. Pour into a glass and serve as a soothing blend of ripe pears and ginger with a gentle texture.

Nutritional Data:
Calories: 150 | Carbohydrates: 36g | Protein: 3g | Fat: 1g | Fiber: 7g | Sugar: 26g

156. Soft Blueberry and Yogurt Drink

Preparation Time: 10 minutes

Ingredients:

- Blueberries
- Plain or vanilla yogurt
- A bit of honey or sugar

Instructions:

1. In a blender, combine blueberries and plain or vanilla yogurt.
2. Add a bit of honey or sugar for sweetness.
3. Blend until the mixture has a slightly textured but soft consistency.
4. Pour into a glass and serve as a nutritious drink blending blueberries and yogurt with a gentle texture.

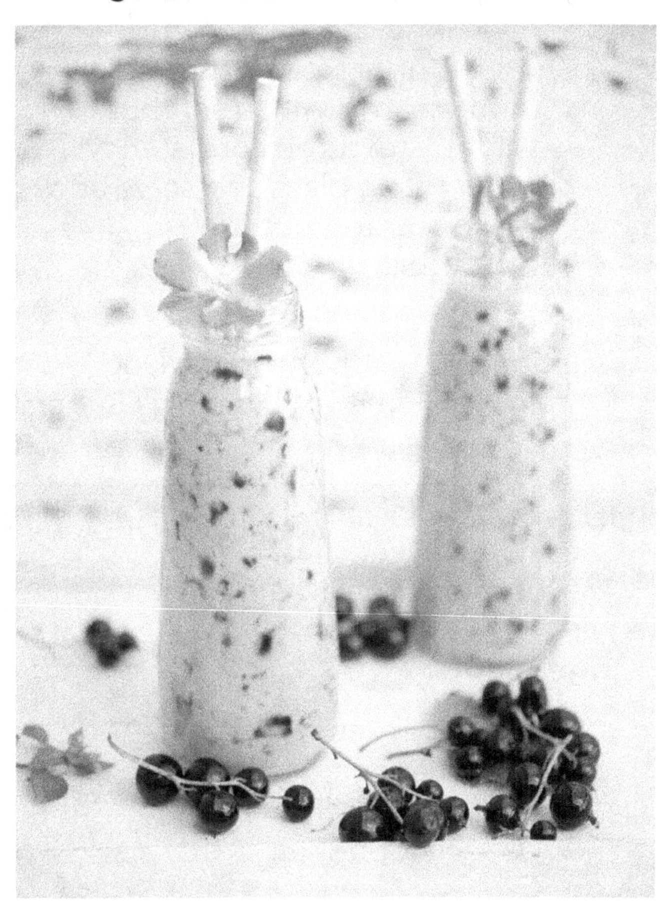

Nutritional Data:
Calories: 120 | Carbohydrates: 25g | Protein: 4g | Fat: 2g | Fiber: 3g | Sugar: 20g

157. Creamy Avocado-Cocoa Smoothie

Preparation Time: 10 minutes

Ingredients:

- Ripe avocado
- Cocoa powder
- Milk or almond milk
- A sweetener like honey or maple syrup

Instructions:

1. Peel and pit the ripe avocado.
2. In a blender, combine the ripe avocado, cocoa powder, milk or almond milk, and a sweetener like honey or maple syrup.
3. Blend until the mixture is rich and creamy, with a soft but slightly textured consistency.
4. Pour into a glass and serve as a delicious and nutritious smoothie.

Nutritional Data:
Calories: 220 | Carbohydrates: 20g | Protein: 4g | Fat: 16g | Fiber: 7g | Sugar: 9g

158. Strawberry-Banana Swirl

Preparation Time: 10 minutes

Ingredients:

- Strawberries
- Ripe banana
- Yogurt or milk
- Honey (optional)

Instructions:

1. In a blender, combine strawberries, ripe bananas, and yogurt or milk.
2. Add honey for sweetness if desired.
3. Blend until the mixture is smooth, with small fruit pieces for texture.
4. Pour into a glass and serve as a classic combination of strawberries and bananas, blended to a smooth consistency.

Nutritional Data:
Calories: 140 | Carbohydrates: 32g | Protein: 4g | Fat: 1g | Fiber: 6g | Sugar: 22g

159. Melon and Mint Refresher

Preparation Time: 10 minutes

Ingredients:

- Cantaloupe or honeydew melon
- Fresh mint leaves
- Water or apple juice

Instructions:

1. Cut the cantaloupe or honeydew melon into small, manageable pieces.
2. Place the melon pieces and fresh mint leaves in a blender.
3. Add a small amount of water or apple juice to facilitate blending.
4. Blend until the mixture is smooth, with a soft texture and small melon pieces remaining.
5. Pour into a glass and serve as a refreshing drink with a hint of mint.

Nutritional Data:
Calories: 80 | Carbohydrates: 20g | Protein: 1g | Fat: 0g | Fiber: 2g | Sugar: 18g

As we come to the close of this culinary journey, I want to extend my heartfelt gratitude to every one of you who has walked this path with us. Your commitment to enhancing the dining experience, regardless of the challenges that dysphagia presents, is truly commendable.

Your health, your satisfaction, and your joy in eating are at the core of why the "Dysphagia Cookbook" was created. It has been an honor to provide you with recipes that we hope have not only nourished your body but also brought pleasure and comfort to your meals.

May the dishes you've discovered and the techniques you've learned serve as steadfast companions on your continued journey toward health improvement. Remember that each bite, each flavor, is a celebration of life and the resilience within you.

I wish you good health, continued progress, and the enduring joy of eating. May your meals always be a source of comfort and a reason to gather, share, and smile.

Thank you for allowing this cookbook to be a part of your table and your journey.

Bon Appétit!

Martha Mc Grew

Thank You!

I hope you enjoyed reading it as much as I enjoyed writing it. _Your support means the world to me!_

If you found value in these pages, I kindly ask you to consider **leaving an honest review on Amazon.** Your feedback not only helps me improve but also helps other readers discover this book.

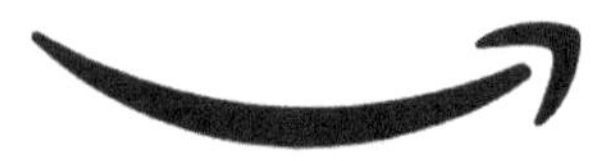

Get access to your bonus!

Download **"Caregiver's Toolkit"**

Scan the QR code
or copy this link: https://o2o.to/i/9IUDIP

...and enjoy your bonus content.